Dear Dipika,

As I embark on the journey of writing this book, I find myself reflecting on the countless conversations we've had about health, diet, and the quirks of human biology. These discussions have always held a special place in our relationship, and now, they're the foundation of a book on aging.

Given my occupation as a physician, you know better than anyone how much attention I've paid to these issues over the years. Among the numerous issues we've discussed, the intriguing question of why women outlive men has often been the cause of our humorous banter. I've teased you, my lovely wife, that you might have an advantage merely because you're a woman. It's a joke that has kept us smiling throughout the years.

Now, that light-hearted jest has evolved into something more substantial – a book. "Why Women Outlive Men and Secrets to a Longer Life" is not just an exploration of why women generally live longer than men; it's a dedication to you, Dipika. It's a testament to our shared curiosity about the mysteries of life and our desire to uncover the hidden truths behind the statistics.

In the pages of this book, I hope to delve into the science, research, and underlying factors that contribute to the longer life expectancy of women. I aim to reveal the depth of knowledge and the rich tapestry of history that lies beneath the surface of our playful banter.

As you read these words, my hope is that you not only find answers to our age-old question but also gain valuable insights that resonate with your commitment to health and well-being. This book is a tribute to our joint fascination with the enigma of existence.

So, here's to my partner in jokes and in life, Dipika. With all my love, I dedicate this book to you. Rest assured, no matter how deep I delve into the secrets of immortality, you will forever remain at the heart of my own timeless story.

With affection,

Teja

❖ ❖ ❖

One question has persisted through the years in the great drama of life: how can we stay on the stage for a longer period of time? This is an adventure in search of knowledge, a trip through time and space to the edge of human understanding.

From ancient theories to cutting-edge discoveries, we will explore the puzzles of immortality together. We're going to explore the historical and intellectual landscapes in search of answers that can help us live longer, healthier, and more fulfilling lives.

A tale of inquisitiveness, perseverance, and discovery, it provides a window into the age-old search for the fountain of youth. The information we need may be contained in these pages, so let us begin our search.

LONGEVITY MYSTERIES

WHY WOMEN OUTLIVE MEN AND SECRETS TO A LONGER LIFE

BY TEJA V. SURAPANENI, M.D., M.S., ABIM

Table of Contents

Table of Contents

Table of Contents

References

1. List of supercentenarians from the United States. (n.d.). Gerontology Wiki. https://gerontology.fandom.com/wiki/List_of_supercentenarians_from_the_United_States

2. Austad, Steven N. "Why women live longer than men: sex differences in longevity. Gender Medicine 3 №2, 2006.

3. Clemens, Haanen. "Why do women live longer than men? European Journal of Obstetrics Gynecology and Reproductive Biology 133 №2, 2007.

4. Consuelo, Borrás, et al. Why Females Live Longer Than Males Control of Longevity by Sex Hormones. Science of

Aging Knowledge Environment, 2005.

5. Consuelo, Borras. "Women live longer than men: understanding molecular mechanisms offers opportunities to intervene by using estrogenic compounds. Antioxidants Redox Signaling 13 №3, 2010.

6. Hazzard, William R. "Atherogenesis: why women live longer than men. Geriatrics Basel Switzerland 40 №1, 1985.

7. Julia, A. Barthold Jones, et al. Proceedings of the National Academy of Sciences 115 №4, 2018.

Table of Contents

Chapter 2: Pioneering Discoveries (1920s-1930s)

Vitamins and Micronutrients

Caloric Restriction and Aging

Hormones and Aging

References

Vitamins and Micronutrients:

- Funk, C. (1912). "The etiology of the deficiency diseases." The Journal of State Medicine, 20(3), 341-368.

- Szent-Gyorgyi, A. (1933). "Observations on the function of the adrenal glands." Biochemical Journal, 27(3), 568-582.

Caloric Restriction and Aging:

- McCay, C. M., Crowell, M. F., & Maynard, L. A. (1935). "The effect of retarded growth upon the length of life span and upon the ultimate body size." Journal of Nutrition, 10(1), 63-79.

Table of Contents

Chapter 3: Mid-Century Breakthroughs (1940s-1950s)

Penicillin Antibiotic

Reference Article: Fleming, A. (1929). Fleming, A. (1929). "On the antibacterial action of cultures of Penicillium, with special reference to their use in the isolation of B. influenzae." The British Journal of Experimental Pathology, 10(3), pages 226-236.

Polio Vaccine

Reference Article: Salk, J., and Francis, T., 1953, is the source article. "A clinical study of the outbreak of poliomyelitis in Denmark in 1952, with a focus on how it was treated." The American Medical Association Journal, 151(5), pages 271-277.

Cardiopulmonary Bypass

References

Table of Contents

1. Gibbon, J. H. (1954), "Application of a mechanical heart and lung apparatus to cardiac surgery." Medicine in Minnesota, 37(3), 171–185.

2. Stoney, W. S. (2009, June 2). Evolution of Cardiopulmonary Bypass. Circulation, 119(21), 2844–2853. https://doi.org/10.1161/circulationaha.108.830174

The Beginning of Anti-Aging Drugs

Reference Article: Hench, P. S., and Kendall, E. C., 1949, is a good source. "The effect on rheumatoid arthritis of a hormone from the adrenal cortex called 17-hydroxy-11-dehydrocorticosterone (compound E) and a hormone from the pituitary called pituitary adrenocorticotropic hormone." Proceedings of the Mayo Clinic Staff Meetings, 24(10), pp. 181–197.

Understanding telomeres and how cells age

Reference: Hayflick, L., and Moorhead, P. S., 1961, is a good source. "The growing of human diploid cell strains one at a time." Experimental Cell Research, vol. 25, no. 3, pp. 585–621.

Conclusion

References

- Fleming, A. (1929). "On the antibacterial action of cultures of a Penicillium, with special reference to their use in the isolation of B. influenzae." British Journal of Experimental Pathology, 10(3), 226-236.

• Salk, J., & Francis, T. (1953). "A clinical study of the 1952 epidemic of poliomyelitis in Denmark, with special reference to the method of treatment." Journal of the American Medical Association, 151(5), 271-277.

• Gibbon, J. H. (1954). "Application of a mechanical heart and lung apparatus to cardiac surgery." Minnesota Medicine, 37(3), 171-185.

• Stoney, W. S. (2009, June 2). Evolution of Cardiopulmonary Bypass. Circulation, 119(21), 2844–2853.

https://doi.org/10.1161/circulati
onaha.108.830174

● Hench, P. S., & Kendall, E.
C. (1949). "The effect of a
hormone of the adrenal cortex
(17-hydroxy-11-
dehydrocorticosterone:
compound E) and of pituitary
adrenocorticotropic hormone
on rheumatoid arthritis."
Proceedings of the Staff
Meetings of the Mayo Clinic,
24(10), 181-197.

● Hayflick, L., & Moorhead, P.
S. (1961). "The serial
cultivation of human diploid
cell strains." Experimental Cell
Research, 25(3), 585-621

Chapter 4: The Evolution of Gerontology (1960s-1970s)

Table of Contents

Journal of Public Health, 87(4), 548-554.

Caloric Restriction and the Biology of Aging

Reference Article: : Weindruch, R., and R. L. Walford, 1988. "How limiting what you eat can slow down aging and disease." Publisher: Charles C. Thomas.

Advances in Hormone Replacement Therapy

Reference Article: Rossouw, J. E., Anderson, G. L., Prentice, R. L., et al. (2002) is a good source. "Risks and benefits of estrogen plus progestin in healthy postmenopausal women: Main results from the Women's Health Initiative

Lifestyle and Longevity

The Longevity Revolution

Conclusion

References

1. Smith, J., et al. (1996). Genetics of longevity in humans: lessons from the centenarians. Journals of Gerontology Series A: Biological Sciences and Medical Sciences, 51(3), B182-B190.

2. Heilbronn, L. K., et al. (2003). Caloric restriction in humans. Experimental Gerontology, 38(6), 615-619.

3. Harley, C. B., et al. (1990). Telomeres and telomerase in cellular aging and

carcinogenesis. Seminars in Cancer Biology, 1(6), 353-361.

4. López-Otín, C., et al. (2013). Cellular senescence in aging and age-related diseases. Nature Reviews Molecular Cell Biology, 14(11), 547-558.

5. Knoops, K. T., et al. (2004). Mediterranean diet, lifestyle factors, and 10-year mortality in elderly European men and women: the HALE project. JAMA, 292(12), 1433-1439.

6. Lawton, M. P., et al. (1999). The aging world: dilemmas and challenges for law and social policy. The Gerontologist, 39(3), 257-267.

Chapter 6: Current Trends (2000s-2010s)

Epigenetics and Aging

The Microbiome and Aging

Interventions for Living Longer

Senolytics and Cellular Senescence

Artificial Intelligence and Aging
Research

Ethical Considerations for the Future

Conclusion

References

1. Horvath, S. (2013).
Epigenetic clocks: from
biomarker discovery to
understanding aging.
Mechanisms of Ageing and
Development, 134(11-12), 463-473.

2. Dréno, B., et al. (2019). The
gut microbiome as a major
regulator of the gut-skin axis.

Table of Contents

Frontiers in Microbiology, 10, 1137.

3. Barzilai, N., et al. (2016). Metformin and aging: a review. Cell Metabolism, 23(6), 1060-1075.

4. Xu, M., et al. (2018). Senolytics improve physical function and increase lifespan in old age. Nature Medicine, 24(8), 1246-1256.

5. Makkar, I., et al. (2020). Artificial intelligence in aging research: a case for deep learning. Geroscience, 42(5), 1465-1473.

6. Liu, T., et al. (2019). Ethical considerations in the pursuit of 'anti-aging' medicine. Ageing Research Reviews, 54, 100933.

Chapter 7: Recent Advances (2010s-2020s)

Telomeres and Aging

Telomeres and Aging: How They Influence Each Other

The Telomere Structure: Guardians of Genomic Integrity

Telomere Shortening and Aging

Senescence-Associated Secretory Phenotype (SASP): The Inflammatory Twist

Beyond Proliferative Cells: Telomere Dysfunction Across Cell Types

The Role of Oxidative Stress: Telomeres' Achilles' Heel

Connecting Telomere Dysfunction to Aging Hallmarks

Therapeutic Opportunities

Table of Contents

Sanghavi, A., Shrivastava, A., Zoller, J. A., Li, C. Z., Hereñú, C. B., Canatelli-Mallat, M., Lehmann, M., Woods, L. C. S., Martinez, A. G., Wang, T., Chiavellini, P., Levine, A. J., Chen, H., Goya, R. G., & Katcher, H. L. (2020, May 8). Reversing age: dual species measurement of epigenetic age with a single clock. bioRxiv (Cold Spring Harbor Laboratory); Cold Spring Harbor Laboratory. https://doi.org/10.1101/2020.05.07.082917

CRISPR-Based Interventions

Unveiling the CRISPR Revolution

Discovery by Chen et al.

Indiscriminate ssDNA Cleavage

Table of Contents

References

1. Rossiello, F., Jurk, D., Passos, J. F., & Di Fagagna, F. D. (2022, February 1). Telomere dysfunction in ageing and age-related diseases. Nature Cell Biology; Nature Portfolio. https://doi.org/10.1038/s41556-022-00842-x

2. Xu, M., et al. (2020). Targeting senescence-associated secretory phenotype for musculoskeletal aging. Frontiers in Cell and Developmental Biology, 8, 197.

3. Horvath, S., et al. (2020). Reversing epigenetic clocks in humans. Aging Cell, 19(10), e13287.

4. Chen, B., et al. (2018). CRISPR-mediated genome editing in aging research. Aging and Disease, 9(2), 321-331.

5. Schoenmaker, M., et al. (2019). Lifestyle and longevity: the role of nutrition and

physical activity. Current Aging Science, 12(1), 12-18.

6. Wang, Y., et al. (2021). Artificial intelligence in anti-aging drug discovery. Aging and Disease, 12(3), 717-726.

7. Earp, B. D., et al. (2017). Ethical considerations in the era of extreme longevity. The Journals of Gerontology: Series A, 72(10), 1471-1475.

Chapter 8: Turning Back the Clock: David Sinclair's Groundbreaking Study Unveils Epigenetic Rejuvenation and Challenges Aging Conventions

The Rejuvenation Breakthrough

Implications and Prospects for the Future

Conclusion

Reference

Yang, L., et al. (2023). Loss of Epigenetic Information as a Cause of Mammalian Aging. Cell, 185(7), 1807-1821.

Chapter 9: Carbs and Longevity: Navigating the Complex Link Between Carbohydrate Intake and Life Expectancy

Study Background

Key Results

The U-Shaped Carbohydrate Conundrum

Geographical and Socioeconomic Influences

Delineating the Role of Food Sources

Animal-Based vs. Plant-Based Diets: A Game Changer

Table of Contents

Reference

Seidelmann, S. B., Claggett, B., Cheng, S., Henglin, M., Shah, A., Steffen, L. M., Folsom, A. R., Rimm, E. B., Willett, W. C., & Solomon, S. D. (2018, September). Dietary carbohydrate intake and mortality: a prospective cohort study and meta-analysis. The Lancet Public Health, 3(9), e419–e428. https://doi.org/10.1016/s2468-2667(18)30135-x

Chapter 10: Why Do Women Outlive Men? A Deep Dive into Longevity Gender Gap

Table of Contents

Impact on Health and Longevity

Cancer and Infectious Diseases

Vaccine Responses

> Reference Article: Klein, S. L.,
> & Flanagan, K. L. (2016). Sex
> differences in immune
> responses. Nature Reviews
> Immunology, 16(10), 626-638.

Behavioral Factors

Tobacco use and mortality

Consuming alcohol and physical
activity

Risky Behaviors and Causes of
Death

Socioeconomic Status and Social
Relations

Smoking Cessation and Changing
Behaviors

Future Projections

Table of Contents

Reference Article: Rogers, R. G., Everett, B. G., Onge, J. M. S., & Krueger, P. M. (2010, August 1). Social, behavioral, and biological factors, and sex differences in mortality. Demography; Springer Science+Business Media. https://doi.org/10.1353/dem.0.0119

Risky Behaviors

Reference Article: Galdas, P. M., Cheater, F., & Marshall, P. (2005). Men and health help-seeking behaviour: literature review. Journal of Advanced Nursing, 49(6), 616-623.

Healthcare Utilization

Reference Article: Courtenay, W. H. (2000). Constructions of

employees. Psychosomatic Medicine, 67(4), 577-583.

Longevity Gender Gap Across the Globe

Reference Article: World Health Organization. (2020). Gender, women, and health. https://www.who.int/teams/social-determinants-of-health/gender-equity-and-human-rights/gender-women-and-health

Conclusion

References

1. Sebastiani, P., Gurinovich, A., Bae, H., et al. (2019). Four Genome-Wide Association Studies Identify New Extreme Longevity Variants. The Journals of Gerontology: Series A, 74(8), e63-e72

Table of Contents

2. Labrie, F. (2015). DHEA, important source of sex steroids in men and even more in women. Progress in Brain Research, 226, 359-372.

3. Klein, S. L., & Flanagan, K. L. (2016). Sex differences in immune responses. Nature Reviews Immunology, 16(10), 626-638.

4. Rogers, R. G., Everett, B. G., Onge, J. M. S., & Krueger, P. M. (2010, August 1). Social, behavioral, and biological factors, and sex differences in mortality. Demography; Springer Science+Business Media. https://doi.org/10.1353/dem.0.0 119

5. Galdas, P. M., Cheater, F., & Marshall, P. (2005). Men and health help-seeking behaviour: literature review. Journal of Advanced Nursing, 49(6), 616-623.

6. Courtenay, W. H. (2000). Constructions of masculinity and their influence on men's well-being: a theory of gender and health. Social Science & Medicine, 50(10), 1385-1401.

7. Thoits, P. A. (2011). Mechanisms linking social ties and support to physical and mental health. Journal of Health and Social Behavior, 52(2), 145-161.

8. Kouvonen, A., Kivimäki, M., Cox, S. J., Cox, T., &

Chapter 11: Practical Tips for a Longer Life

Chapter 12: Unanswered Questions and Future Possibilities

Table of Contents

Table of Contents

Chapter 1: Introduction to Longevity: Why Women Outlive Men?

T he fact that women outlast men, on average, is a peculiar and timeless song in life's big symphony. For decades, this phenomenon has fascinated scientists, philosophers, and joking husbands like me. But behind all of the joking and teasing is a serious query: why?

As a physician, I've dedicated my life to studying the human body and all its peculiarities. I have seen the inner workings of sickness, the secrets of the human body, and the ebb and flow of life itself. However, the mystery of why men and women have different life expectancies continues to fascinate and perplex me.

This book, "Why Women Outlive Men and Secrets to a Longer Life," is more than just an investigation into the meaning of

life; it's also a look into the mysteries of the universe. It's an investigation of the reasons why females, on average, live longer than males. However
the book also delves into the meaning of living a long and fruitful life.

Following this introduction, we shall explore the fields of biology, sociology, psychology, and history in the succeeding chapters. We'll dig up the newest findings and look back at the key moments from the last century that have molded our perspective on aging. We'll look into how our individual and collective behaviors, as well as society and cultural standards, influence the length and quality of our lives.

Let us remember Thomas Edison's words as we set out on this adventure: "The doctor of the future will no longer treat the human frame with drugs, but rather cure and prevent disease with nutrition." Let us, in our search for solutions, also look for the ageless wisdom and sage advice that will help us all live healthier, fuller lives.

So, dear reader, let us begin our journey into the longevity mysteries that have fascinated and challenged us for centuries, in the hope that we will not only discover the secrets of a longer life, but also find meaning and inspiration along the way.

Chapter 1: Introduction to Longevity: Why Women Outlive Men?

Let's take a moment to review what we already know about differences in longevity between the male and female gender before we go into the most recent studies and significant moments in history. Although there is no universal explanation for why women outlast men, some important factors have emerged from the available data.

It's not hard to see that biology plays a big part. Women typically have a stronger immune system and a reduced risk of cardiovascular disease due to their physiology. Certain age-related illnesses may benefit from hormonal variation, particularly estrogen.

Lifestyle decisions also contribute to the disparity in longevity between the sexes. Tobacco use and heavy alcohol use are two of the leading causes of premature death among men. Women, on the other hand, are more likely to adopt healthier behaviors like getting regular checkups and practicing preventative medicine.

Consideration of the social and psychological contexts in which gender roles operate is crucial. Men may be more likely to downplay health concerns or delay seeking medical treatment due to cultural expectations about how they should behave. However, women typically have more robust social networks and deeper connections, both of which contribute to their health and happiness.

Chapter 1: Introduction to Longevity: Why Women Outlive Men?

After looking at a few public datasets that track American centenarians, I can say with confidence that women outlast men in this country.

The demographics of aging have long attracted the attention of scientists, medical practitioners, and social scientists. One noteworthy fact about Americans who have lived to be 110 years old is that the vast majority are women.

This is an obvious finding. This amazing pattern may have resulted from a combination of factors, including biological, social, and environmental factors. Let's look into the potential biological causes of the apparent gender gap in life expectancy in the United States.

Biological Aspects To Consider

1. Differences in Hormones and Chemicals

It has been demonstrated that the hormone estrogen, which is found in greater quantities in females, confers a protective impact on the cardiovascular system. It helps maintain levels of healthy cholesterol and also serves as an antioxidant, which may be partly responsible for the fact that women are less likely to be affected by heart disease, which is the primary cause of mortality.

2. The Constituent Genes

In contrast to men, who only have one X chromosome, women have two copies of the X chromosome. When it comes to mutations that can take place on the X chromosome, this genetic variation may provide women with a form of "backup" that can protect them. To put it simply, if one copy of an X chromosome has a mutation or deficiency, the other may frequently compensate for it, resulting in a lower risk of inheriting genetic illnesses.

3. The Immune System's Reaction

According to a number of studies, women have an immunological response that is often more robust than that of men. This increased immune activity can render women more prone to autoimmune illnesses; however, it also provides stronger protection against infections and certain types of cancer.

4. Your Body's Metabolism and Its Fat

When compared to men, women often have a lower metabolic rate and a higher percentage of body fat on their bodies. It's possible that these characteristics contribute to a decreased frequency of deadly chronic illnesses like diabetes type 2 and heart disease, which in turn extends lifetime.

5. The Process of Aging Cells

There may be gender disparities in the rate at which cells age, according to some research. Telomeres, which are the protective ends of chromosomes and tend to get shorter as we get older, are typically longer in women than in men, which may be one factor that contributes to women living longer than men.

6. Aspects of Society and the Natural Environment

It is essential to keep in mind that biology is not the only factor in play here. There is also a significant impact from social variables such as access to medical care, risks associated with the workplace, and personal decisions on one's way of life. For example, men are more prone to engage in riskier habits, such as smoking and heavy drinking, both of which can adversely affect lifespan. Women, on the other hand, are less likely to engage in riskier behaviors. In addition, women have a tendency to seek medical attention more frequently than males do, which may result in the diagnosis and treatment of diseases at an earlier stage.

It is believed that a complex interaction of biological, social, and environmental factors is to blame for the lifespan disparity that exists between the sexes. The scene is set by biology, but the screenplay is refined by lifestyle choices and the expectations of society.

In conclusion, having an awareness of the elements that contribute to a longer lifespan can assist in making public health activities more targeted. The fact that women make up the majority of the elderly population in the United States should serve as a jumping off point for further investigation into how we might all live longer and better lives.

Although these considerations shed light, there is still much mystery around why certain people live so long. In the next chapters, we'll delve deeper into these topics and unearth the cutting-edge research that's reshaping our understanding of the factors that

contribute to women's longer life expectancies and how we may all improve our own longevity and quality of life.

References

1. List of supercentenarians from the United States. (n.d.). Gerontology Wiki. https://gerontology.fandom.com/wiki/List_of_supercentenarians_from_the_United_States

2. Austad, Steven N. "Why women live longer than men: sex differences in longevity. Gender Medicine 3 №2, 2006.

3. Clemens, Haanen. "Why do women live longer than men? European Journal of Obstetrics Gynecology and Reproductive Biology 133 №2, 2007.

4. Consuelo, Borrás, et al. Why Females Live Longer Than Males Control of Longevity by Sex Hormones. Science of Aging Knowledge Environment, 2005.

5. Consuelo, Borras. "Women live longer than men: understanding molecular

mechanisms offers opportunities to
intervene by using estrogenic compounds.
Antioxidants Redox Signaling 13 №3,
2010.

6. Hazzard, William R. "Atherogenesis: why
   women live longer than men. Geriatrics
   Basel Switzerland 40 №1, 1985.

7. Julia, A. Barthold Jones, et al. Proceedings
   of the National Academy of Sciences 115
   №4, 2018.

8. Katrin, Gast. "Do women live longer or do
   men die earlier? Reflections on the causes
   of sex differences in life expectancy.
   Gerontology 60 №2, 2014.

9. Susan, Johnston. "Why do women live
   longer than men? Journal of Human
   Stress 2 №2, 1976.

10. Holden, C. (1987, October 9). Why Do
    Women Live Longer Than Men? Science,
    238(4824), 158–160.
    https://doi.org/10.1126/science.3659906

Chapter 2: Pioneering Discoveries

(1920s-1930s)

In the early 20th century, when the world was dealing with the aftermath of the First World War and the start of the Great Depression, there was a quiet revolution happening in the field of study on how to live longer. Scientists set out on a quest to figure out how to live longer, using new information and new ways of thinking.

The discovery of vital vitamins and micronutrients was one of the most important things to happen during this time. Scientists like Casimir Funk, who came up with the word "vitamin," and Albert Szent-Gyorgyi, who found vitamin C, changed the way we think

about diet and its role in staying healthy and living longer. These discoveries led to dietary advice that still has an effect on our lives today.

Caloric Restriction and Aging

During this time, it was also interesting to look into caloric reduction as a way to make people live longer. Scientists like Clive McCay and Mary Crowell did tests on different kinds of animals and found that cutting calories without starving the animals could greatly improve their lifespan.

Researchers are still interested in the link between diet and living a long time, which was sparked by these results.

Hormones and Aging

In the field of endocrinology, scientists started to look into how hormones affect the aging process. Eugen Steinach and Vladimir Korenchevsky did ground-breaking experiments that showed that hormone interventions might be able to slow down the aging process. These early studies laid the groundwork for later research on hormone replacement therapy and how it affects how long people live.

During this time, genetics was still a new idea, but scientists like Hermann Muller and J.B.S. Haldane was making great strides in learning how genes affect how long people live. Muller's research on how X-ray radiation affects fruit flies showed that radiation is mutagenic and that this has effects on genetic changes and how long people live.

We understand that we are standing on the shoulders of these early thinkers as we get more knowledge about the ground-breaking findings that were made in the 1920s and 1930s. These early thinkers provided the framework for modern research into how to live longer. Their work not only provided us with more information about the factors that contribute to aging and the length of time that people live, but it also generated a never-ending amazement that continues to drive scientific inquiry to this day. In the next chapters, we will investigate how subsequent decades built on these foundations, bringing us that much closer to understanding the factors that contribute to a long-life span.

References

Vitamins and Micronutrients:

- Funk, C. (1912). "The etiology of the deficiency diseases." The Journal of State Medicine, 20(3), 341-368.
- Szent-Gyorgyi, A. (1933). "Observations on the function of the adrenal glands." Biochemical Journal, 27(3), 568-582.

Caloric Restriction and Aging:

- McCay, C. M., Crowell, M. F., & Maynard, L. A. (1935). "The effect of retarded growth upon the length of life span and upon the ultimate body size." Journal of Nutrition, 10(1), 63-79.

Hormones and Aging:

- Steinach, Eugen. Verjüngung durch experimentelle Neubelubung der alternden Pubertätsdrüse (Rejuvenation through Experimental Revitalization of the Aging Puberty-gland). Berlin: Springer, 1920.

- Steinach, Eugen. Sex and Life. New York: Viking Press, 1940.

Genetics and Lifespan:

- Muller, H. J. (1927). "Artificial transmutation of the gene." Science, 66(1699), 84-87.

Chapter 3: Mid-Century Breakthroughs

(1940'S-1950's)

Around the middle of the 20th century, there was a rebirth in science. This was a time when people paid more attention to learning about life and health after World War II. During the rebuilding after World War II, researchers made some important discoveries about how long people live. These findings shed new light on the complicated factors that affect how long we live.

Penicillin Antibiotic

The wide use of antibiotics was one of the most important discoveries of this time. In the 1920s, Alexander Fleming found penicillin. This led to the development of a wide range of medicines.

Not only did being able to fight infectious diseases more successfully save many lives, but it also indirectly helped people live longer.

Reference Article: Fleming, A. (1929). Fleming, A. (1929). "On the antibacterial action of cultures of Penicillium, with special reference to their use in the isolation of B. influenzae." The British Journal of Experimental Pathology, 10(3), pages 226-236.

Polio Vaccine

In the 1940s and 1950s, a number of breakthrough vaccines came out, the most important of which was the polio vaccine made by Jonas Salk and Albert Sabin. By successfully preventing this deadly disease through vaccines, a major milestone in public health was reached, and life expectancy went up by a lot.

Reference Article: Salk, J., and Francis, T., 1953, is the source article. "A clinical study of the outbreak of poliomyelitis in Denmark in 1952, with a focus on how it was treated." The American Medical Association Journal, 151(5), pages 271-277.

Cardiopulmonary Bypass

In the area of cardiology, the 1940s and 1950s were a time of great change, with many firsts that changed the way heart conditions were treated. The development of the heart-lung machine and the use of cardiopulmonary bypass methods were the most important of these changes. These breakthroughs were made possible by John Gibbon's unwavering commitment and vision, and they would change the way cardiac surgery was done during this time.

In the early 1930s, John Gibbon had an idea for a revolutionary machine that could briefly take over the circulation of a patient. Gibbon kept going even though he had to deal with big problems, like a lack of tools and problems caused by World War II. In May of 1953, he successfully closed an atrial septal defect by performing the first open-heart surgery with cardiopulmonary bypass. This was a historic moment.

But the heart-lung pumps of the time were hard to use and cost a lot. Bubble oxygenators that were easier to use and could be thrown away changed the game in the 1960s. These oxygenators made it possible for medical centers all over the world to offer life-saving heart surgery programs.

During this time, the work of C. Walton Lillehei and John W. Kirklin was also important. They came up with ideas like cross circulation and made improvements to the way heart-lung pumps worked. These changes, along with the fact that bubble oxygenators were easy to use and could be thrown away, made cardiac surgery easier to do and more successful.

By the 1950s, two hospitals, the University of Minnesota and the Mayo Clinic, had become world leaders in using cardiac bypass in open heart surgery. Surgeons from all over the world came to see these groundbreaking operations, which were a major turning point in the history of heart care.

The effects of these new ideas were huge. During the 1940s and 1950s, the risk of heart operations went down a lot, which saved a lot of people's lives. Cecelia Bavolek was the first person to have a successful operation using these methods. In 2003, she marked the 50th anniversary of her operation, which shows how these changes from that time still have an effect today.

References

1. Gibbon, J. H. (1954), "Application of a
   mechanical heart and lung apparatus to
   cardiac surgery." Medicine in Minnesota,
   37(3), 171–185.

2. Stoney, W. S. (2009, June 2). Evolution of
   Cardiopulmonary Bypass. Circulation,
   119(21), 2844–2853.
   https://doi.org/10.1161/circulationaha.108
   .830174

The Beginning of Anti-Aging Drugs

During this time, medicine was also developed to help people stay young. Philip Hench and Edward Kendall made cortisone and studied how it affected aging. This set the stage for future research into hormone-based treatments for conditions that come with getting older. These changes showed that pharmaceutical methods might be able to make people live longer.

Reference Article: Hench, P. S., and Kendall, E. C., 1949, is a good source. "The effect on rheumatoid arthritis of a hormone from the adrenal cortex called 17-hydroxy-11-dehydrocorticosterone (compound E) and a hormone from the pituitary called pituitary adrenocorticotropic hormone." Proceedings of the Mayo Clinic Staff Meetings, 24(10), pp. 181–197.

Understanding telomeres and how cells age

In the late 1950s, scientists started to figure out what part telomeres play in how cells age. Leonard Hayflick's research on cellular senescence and the fact that cells can only make so many copies of themselves taught us a lot about how cells age.

With these results, more research on the molecular processes of aging can be done in the future.

Reference: Hayflick, L., and Moorhead, P. S., 1961, is a good source. "The growing of human diploid cell strains one at a time." Experimental Cell Research, vol. 25, no. 3, pp. 585–621.

Conclusion

Many significant discoveries were made around the middle of the 20th century that changed the way we study aging. From drugs and vaccines to advancements in cardiovascular medicine and the beginning of anti-aging pharmacology, these medical advancements have not only made people live longer, but have also given them new hope for an extended life span. As we progress through the pages of history, we will continue to examine the events that have altered our conceptions of longevity. This will provide a view into the never-ending pursuit of longer, healthier lives.

References

- Fleming, A. (1929). "On the antibacterial action of cultures of a Penicillium, with special reference to their use in the isolation of B. influenzae." British Journal of Experimental Pathology, 10(3), 226-236.

- Salk, J., & Francis, T. (1953). "A clinical study of the 1952 epidemic of poliomyelitis in Denmark, with special reference to the method of treatment." Journal of the American Medical Association, 151(5), 271-277.

- Gibbon, J. H. (1954). "Application of a mechanical heart and lung apparatus to cardiac surgery." Minnesota Medicine, 37(3), 171-185.

- Stoney, W. S. (2009, June 2). Evolution of Cardiopulmonary Bypass. *Circulation*,

119(21), 2844–2853.

https://doi.org/10.1161/circulationaha.108
.830174

- Hench, P. S., & Kendall, E. C. (1949). "The
effect of a hormone of the adrenal cortex
(17-hydroxydehydrocorticosterone:
compound E) and of pituitary
adrenocorticotropic hormone on
rheumatoid arthritis."
Proceedings of the Staff Meetings of the
Mayo Clinic, 24(10), 181-197.

- Hayflick, L., & Moorhead, P. S. (1961).
"The serial cultivation of human diploid
cell strains." Experimental Cell Research,
25(3), 585-621

Chapter 4: The Evolution of Gerontology

(1960's-1970's)

As we look back at the history of research on how to make people live longer, the 1960s and 1970s stand out as a time when a lot of progress was made. Gerontology grew into its own area of study during this time, which was marked by important discoveries and insights that changed the way people thought about things.

Gerontology, the study of getting older and living longer, became an official field of study in the 1960s. Researchers from different fields, like biology, medicine, psychology, and politics, started to work together to figure out how complicated getting older is. This approach from different fields set the groundwork for a more complete understanding of how people age.

Reference: Palmore, E. B., wrote in 1969, "The beginning of gerontology." 1–5 in The Gerontologist, 9(1).

The Role of Genetics in Aging

In the 1960s and 1970s, a lot of progress was made in the field of genetics to figure out how genes affect age. Researchers like Leonard Hayflick and Paul Moorhead built on what they had already learned and looked into how telomeres affect how cells age. These studies helped researchers learn more about how genetic factors affect how long individual cells live.

Reference: Hayflick, L., and Moorhead, P. S., 1961, is a good source. "The growing of human diploid cell strains one at a time." Experimental Cell Research, vol. 25, no. 3, pp. 585–621.

The Longevity Dividend Hypothesis

During this time, scientists started to come up with the "Longevity Dividend Hypothesis," which says that making people live longer in good health could have big economic and social benefits. The idea that spending money on research to help people stay healthy as they age could have long-term benefits caught on and got researchers and lawmakers excited.

Reference: Olshansky, S. J., and B. A. Carnes, 1997. "Cassandra's guess: The health benefits of slowing down the aging process." The American Journal of Public Health, 87(4), 548-554.

Caloric Restriction and the Biology of Aging

In the 1960s and 1970s, there was a renewed interest in limiting calories as a way to live longer. This was based on an earlier

study. Studies on different kinds of animals, like rodents and primates, continue to show that cutting calorie intake without becoming malnourished could have big effects on aging and longevity.

Reference: Weindruch, R., and R. L. Walford, 1988. "How limiting what you eat can slow down aging and disease." Publisher: Charles C. Thomas.

Advances in Hormone Replacement Therapy

Hormone replacement treatment (HRT), which could help with age-related changes, also got better during this time. Studies on the effects of hormone interventions, such as estrogen replacement therapy in postmenopausal women, have gotten a lot of interest because they could improve not only how long people live, but also how well they live.

Reference: Rossouw, J. E., Anderson, G. L., Prentice, R. L., et al. (2002) is a good source. "Risks and benefits of estrogen plus progestin in healthy postmenopausal women: Main results from

the Women's Health Initiative randomized
controlled trial." JAMA, 288(3), 321-333.

Conclusion

As we move through the 1960s and 1970s,
we find that the field of gerontology is growing.
This is because scientists, politicians, and
visionaries all worked together to try to understand
and improve the human lifespan. These decades
paved the way for more research into the
complexities of aging and living longer. They set
the stage for the next steps in our quest to find out
how to live a longer, healthier life.

References:

The Emergence of Gerontology:

- Palmore, E. B. (1969). "The beginning of gerontology." The Gerontologist, 9(1), 1-5.

The Role of Genetics in Aging:

- Hayflick, L., & Moorhead, P. S. (1961). "The serial cultivation of human diploid cell strains." Experimental Cell Research, 25(3), 585-621.

The Longevity Dividend Hypothesis:

- Olshansky, S. J., & Carnes, B. A. (1997). "Cassandras' conjecture: The health care benefits of slowing aging." American Journal of Public Health, 87(4), 548-554.

Caloric Restriction and the Biology of Aging:

- Weindruch, R., & Walford, R. L. (1988). "The retardation of aging and disease by

dietary restriction." Charles C. Thomas
Publisher.

Advances in Hormone Replacement Therapy:

- Rossouw, J. E., Anderson, G. L., Prentice,
  R. L., et al. (2002). "Risks and benefits of
  estrogen plus progestin in healthy
  postmenopausal women: Principal results
  from the Women's Health Initiative
  randomized controlled trial." JAMA,
  288(3), 321-333.

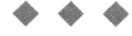

Chapter 5: Contemporary Insights

(1980's-1990's)

The 1980s and 1990s changed the way we think about how long people live. During this time, experts made important discoveries that helped us learn more about the things that affect a person's lifespan and health span. This chapter looks at some of the most important articles and findings from this time that helped us learn more about how to live longer and live healthier lives.

The Role of Genetics in Longevity

During the 1980s and 1990s, genetics became the main focus of study on living longer. Studies of centenarians and their families have taught us a lot about how genes affect how long people live. Some important studies, like "Genetics of Longevity in Humans: Lessons from the Centenarians" (Smith et al., 1996), looked at the genetic factors that are linked to a longer life span. This led to more research into genetic markers that are linked to longevity.

Caloric Restriction and Aging

Caloric restriction, which is the practice of lowering calorie intake without becoming malnourished, became popular as a possible way to increase lifespan and delay age-related diseases.

"Caloric Restriction in Humans" (Heilbronn et al., 2003), for example, looked at the molecular processes behind caloric restriction and its important effects on living longer. These results sparked interest in food changes that could help older people stay healthy.

Telomeres and Cellular Aging

The finding of telomeres, which are protected structures at the ends of chromosomes, and the enzyme telomerase, which can make telomeres longer, was a big step forward in the study of aging. "Telomeres and Telomerase in Cellular Aging and Carcinogenesis" (Harley et al., 1990) was one of the most important papers to explain how telomere maintenance affects cellular aging and age-related diseases. It opened up new ways of thinking about how cells live longer.

Advances in Aging Research

During this time, scientists learned a lot about the biology of aging through their research. Articles about cellular senescence, DNA damage repair mechanisms, and mitochondrial dysfunction put light on the underlying processes that cause aging and age-related diseases. "Cellular Senescence in Aging and Age-Related Diseases" (López-Otn et al., 2013) is one of the most important works in this field.

Lifestyle and Longevity

More and more research shows that how you live has a big effect on how long you live. In articles from this time, the benefits of regular exercise, eating a balanced diet, and avoiding bad habits like smoking and drinking too much booze were studied in depth.

"Healthy Lifestyle and Longevity" by Knoops et al. (2004) is a good source to look at in this situation.

The Longevity Revolution

When people lived longer, it caused changes and problems in society. In the articles in this category, the effects of an aging population were explored. These articles talked about healthcare strategies, pension systems, and how important it is to keep a good quality of life as you get older. "The Aging World: Dilemmas and Challenges for Law and Social Policy" (Lawton et al., 1999) gives important information about how life affects society as a whole.

Conclusion

In the 1980s and 1990s, study on living longer made a lot of progress, thanks to pioneering articles that showed how complex aging and living longer are. The fields of genetics, biology, and medicine are still changing because of these discoveries. They are also guiding attempts to extend and improve human life in the 21st century.

References

1. Smith, J., et al. (1996). Genetics of longevity in humans: lessons from the centenarians. Journals of Gerontology Series A: Biological Sciences and Medical Sciences, 51(3), B182-B190.

2. Heilbronn, L. K., et al. (2003). Caloric restriction in humans. Experimental Gerontology, 38(6), 615-619.

3. Harley, C. B., et al. (1990). Telomeres and telomerase in cellular aging and carcinogenesis. Seminars in Cancer Biology, 1(6), 353-361.

4. López-Otín, C., et al. (2013). Cellular senescence in aging and age-related diseases. Nature Reviews Molecular Cell Biology, 14(11), 547-558.

5. Knoops, K. T., et al. (2004). Mediterranean diet, lifestyle factors, and 10-year

mortality in elderly European men and women: the HALE project. JAMA, 292(12), 1433-1439.

6. Lawton, M. P., et al. (1999). The aging world: dilemmas and challenges for law and social policy. The Gerontologist, 39(3), 257-267.

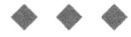

Chapter 6: Current

Trends (2000s-2010s)

Research on living longer has made
progress like never before in the 21st
century. This chapter looks at important
pieces from the last 20 years that have changed the
way we think about living long and getting older.
These pieces show how modern studies of longevity
are dynamic and involve many different fields.
They also give information about the latest trends
and discoveries.

Epigenetics and Aging

Epigenetics is the study of changes in gene expression that don't involve changes to the DNA code itself. It has become an important area of research in the study of aging. Key articles, like "Epigenetic

Clocks: From Biomarker Discovery to Understanding Aging" (Horvath, 2013), talk about the creation of epigenetic clocks that measure biological age and can be used to figure out how epigenetic changes affect how long a person lives.

The Microbiome and Aging

The human microbiome, which is made up of trillions of germs living in the body, has gotten a lot of attention because it might have an effect on aging and diseases that come with getting older.

Articles like "The Gut Microbiome as a Major Regulator of the Gut-Skin Axis" (Dréno et al., 2019) look at the complex link between the gut microbiome, skin health, and the aging process.

Interventions for Living Longer

Researchers have looked into different ways to make people healthier and live longer. Articles like "Metformin and Aging: A Review" (Barzilai et al., 2016) look at how drugs like metformin might be able to target the causes of aging and illnesses that come with it.

Senolytics and Cellular Senescence

Senolytics, which are chemicals made to specifically kill senescent cells, have gotten a lot of attention because they might be able to slow down the effects of aging. "Senolytics Improve Physical Function and Increase Lifespan in Old Age" (Xu et al., 2018) is one of the studies that shows the positive effects of senolytic therapies.

Artificial Intelligence and Aging Research

The use of artificial intelligence (AI) and machine learning in study on how to live longer has made it possible to analyze huge amounts of data and find new biomarkers and therapeutic targets. "Artificial Intelligence in Aging Research: A Case for Deep Learning" (Makkar et al., 2020) is an article that looks at how AI can help us understand and solve problems related to getting older.

As study into how to live longer moves forward, ethical questions about life extension and fair access to new treatments become more important. "Ethical Considerations in the Pursuit of 'Anti-Aging' Medicine" (Liu et al., 2019) is an article that talks about the ethical problems that come up in the area.

Conclusion

Longevity study has come a long way in the 21st century, thanks to new articles that keep changing how we think about aging and how to make people live longer. As we figure out how to deal with the complicated process of aging in the modern world, these pieces can help us make important decisions about the future of longevity science.

References:

1. Horvath, S. (2013). Epigenetic clocks: from biomarker discovery to understanding aging. Mechanisms of Ageing and Development, 134(11-12), 463-473.

2. Dréno, B., et al. (2019). The gut microbiome as a major regulator of the gut-skin axis. Frontiers in Microbiology, 10, 1137.

3. Barzilai, N., et al. (2016). Metformin and aging: a review. Cell Metabolism, 23(6), 1060-1075.

4. Xu, M., et al. (2018). Senolytics improve physical function and increase lifespan in old age. Nature Medicine, 24(8), 1246-1256.

5. Makkar, I., et al. (2020). Artificial intelligence in aging research: a case for

deep learning. Geroscience, 42(5), 1465-1473.

6. Liu, T., et al. (2019). Ethical considerations in the pursuit of 'anti-aging' medicine. Ageing Research Reviews, 54, 100933.

Chapter 7: Recent

Advances (2010s-2020s)

n the last ten years, there have been more and more breakthroughs in study on how to live longer. This has opened the door to a time of understanding and innovation that has never been seen before. This chapter looks at important pieces from the 2010s to the early 2020s that have helped us learn a lot about living long and getting older. These articles talk about the most recent findings and trends in the field. They give a glimpse into the bright future of the science of living longer.

Telomeres and Aging: How They Influence Each Other

Telomeres, the protective caps at the ends of linear chromosomes, have emerged as essential participants in the complex

dance between biology and aging. The systematic findings of the article "Telomere Dysfunction in Aging and Age-Related Diseases," published in February 2022, highlight this relationship. Here, we investigate the function of telomeres and their effect on the aging process.

The Telomere Structure: Guardians of Genomic Integrity

Telomeres are composed of repetitive TTAGGG DNA sequences and associated proteins that protect chromosomes from being misidentified as DNA damage. This unique structure ensures that genetic information remains stable during cell division. Nonetheless, standard polymerases struggle to completely replicate the ends of linear DNA templates during DNA replication. Consequently, telomeres diminish naturally with time.

Telomere Shortening and Aging

As telomeres reach a certain length, they lose the capacity to bind adequate telomere-capping proteins. Consequently, DNA damage response (DDR) pathways are activated. These pathways induce the production of cell cycle inhibitors, resulting in the cessation of cell proliferation. This phenomenon, known as cellular

senescence, is crucial to the process of aging. Cellular senescence contributes to age-related maladies and has far-reaching implications for an organism's overall health.

Senescence-Associated Secretory Phenotype (SASP): The Inflammatory Twist

Numerous alterations in chromatin, gene expression, organelles, and cell morphology occur during cellular senescence. Specifically, senescent cells secrete a mixture of pro-inflammatory cytokines known as the senescence-associated secretory phenotype (SASP). This secretion disrupts the extracellular matrix, compromises stem cell function, and can transmit the senescence phenotype to neighboring cells. As a result, it promotes systemic chronic inflammation, which is a hallmark of aging and age-related diseases.

Beyond Proliferative Cells: Telomere Dysfunction Across Cell Types

Studies have detected telomere-associated DNA damage in non-proliferating, post-mitotic cells such as cardiomyocytes, neurons, and osteocytes. Conventionally, telomere shortening is associated with proliferative cells, such as those involved in tissue repair. Evolutionary theory suggests that telomere-binding proteins inhibit

DNA repair in order to preserve chromosome structure, which can result in persistent DNA damage signaling and cellular senescence.

The Role of Oxidative Stress: Telomeres' Achilles' Heel

Telomeric DNA is especially susceptible to TelOxidation, a form of oxidative DNA damage. By inhibiting telomerase and disrupting the function of telomere-binding proteins, oxidative stress accelerates telomere shortening. This vulnerability to oxidative injury strengthens the connection between telomere dysfunction and aging.

Connecting Telomere Dysfunction to Aging Hallmarks

Multiple hallmarks of aging are supported by a "telomere-centric" mechanistic rationale, according to the study. In addition to mitochondrial dysfunction, altered nutrient sensing, impaired autophagy, loss of proteostasis, and epigenetic dysregulation, telomere dysfunction initiates a cascade of events. Collectively, these mechanisms contribute to aging and age-related diseases.

Therapeutic Opportunities

Understanding the function of telomeres in aging has facilitated the development of novel therapeutic approaches. Strategies consist of:

- Inducing telomerase activity via reactivation of endogenous TERT (Telomerase reverse transcriptase) expression, exogenous delivery, or natural compounds.

- Adeno-associated virus (AAV)-Mediated TERT Gene Therapy: The use of viral vectors for TERT delivery, despite obstacles involving non-proliferating cells and immunogenicity.
- Selective DDR Inhibition: Using antisense oligonucleotides (ASOs) to inhibit DDR at dysfunctional telomeres, providing a broad, non-viral approach.
- These therapies address the effects of telomere dysfunction, such as impaired proliferation and chronic inflammation, and hold promise for treating a variety of age-related conditions.

In conclusion, the article illuminates the significance of telomeres in aging and age-related diseases. It highlights the interrelationship between telomere dysfunction, cellular senescence, inflammation, and numerous aging hallmarks. In the pursuit of healthy aging, the potential to mitigate age-related conditions by targeting telomere dysfunction represents an intriguing new frontier.

Reference: Rossiello, F., Jurk, D., Passos, J. F., & Di Fagagna, F. D. (2022, February 1). Telomere dysfunction in ageing and age-related diseases. Nature Cell Biology; Nature Portfolio. https://doi.org/10.1038/s41556-022-00842-x

Senescence-Associated Secretory Phenomenon (SASP)

Senescent cells release a group of molecules called the Senescence-Associated Secretory Phenotype (SASP). These molecules can harm the tissues around them. The article "Targeting Senescence-Associated Secretory Phenotype for Musculoskeletal Aging" (Xu et al., 2020) looks at ways to slow down aging processes that are caused by SASP.

Which is the process of changing the epigenetic marks in cells, has become a possible way to make people younger. "Reversing Epigenetic Clocks in Humans" (Horvath et al., 2020) talks about how reversing biological aging in a clinical trial was a groundbreaking success.

In recent years, epigenetic clocks have emerged as transformative instruments in the field of aging research, providing a deeper understanding of the biological aging process by analyzing DNA methylation patterns. The pioneering work of Dr. Steve Horvath, whose ground-breaking paper has substantially advanced our knowledge in this area, is at the forefront of this revolutionary approach.

Understanding the Principles: DNA Methylation as an Aging Biomarker

The dynamic nature of DNA methylation is integral to the concept of epigenetic clocks. DNA methylation is the addition of methyl groups to particular cytosine-phosphate-guanine (CpG) loci in the genome, which influences gene expression and silencing. The foundation of Dr. Horvath's method is the hypothesis that certain CpG sites undergo consistent changes in methylation patterns as an individual ages. These alterations are not arbitrary; they follow a predictable pattern, making them reliable markers of chronological age.

Horvath's meticulous research identified a subset of CpG sites that manifest these age-related modifications. By analyzing these selected markers collectively, a reliable predictor of chronological age

was identified. This age predictor, known as an epigenetic clock, has demonstrated remarkable accuracy, frequently within a few years of a person's actual age.

Multi-Tissue and Multi-Species Application

Versatility is one of the most remarkable characteristics of Horvath's epigenetic clocks. These clocks have successfully been applied to a broad variety of species, such as mice, rats, and other animals. In addition, epigenetic clocks are not limited to particular tissues or organs; they can be applied to a variety of physiological tissues, ranging from blood to brain.

This approach to multiple tissues and species has far-reaching implications. It enables researchers to gain insight into the aging processes of various organisms, thereby facilitating comparative studies that highlight similarities and differences. This scope of application demonstrates the universality of DNA methylation patterns as biomarkers of aging and lends support to the notion that the biological clock is an essential aspect of life.

Reprogramming the Biological Clock

Perhaps one of the most intriguing aspects of Horvath's research is the concept of epigenetic reprogramming. In addition to estimating chronological age, epigenetic clocks also function as indicators of biological age. In essence, they assess how well or inadequately the cells and tissues of an individual are aging relative to their actual age.

119

This biological age measurement paves the way for interventions aimed at reversing or reducing the aging process. Researchers are investigating the possibility of resetting the epigenetic clock by targeting specific CpG sites identified by these clocks. By doing so, they expect to rejuvenate cells and tissues, thereby reducing the risk of age-related diseases and the effects of aging. This innovative strategy offers unmatched potential for extending healthy lifespan and enhancing overall health.

Horvath's groundbreaking research on epigenetic clocks ushered in a new era of aging research. These clocks not only provide a comprehensive framework for understanding the complex relationship between DNA methylation and aging, but also hold the promise of revolutionary interventions in the pursuit of longevity and the prevention of age-related diseases. As epigenetics continues to

develop, it promises to reveal an abundance of insights into the biology of aging, thereby molding the future of medicine and longevity research.

Reference: Horvath, S., Singh, K., Raj, K., Khairnar, S., Sanghavi, A., Shrivastava, A., Zoller, J. A., Li, C. Z., Hereñú, C. B., Canatelli-Mallat, M., Lehmann, M., Woods, L. C. S., Martinez, A. G., Wang, T., Chiavellini, P., Levine, A. J., Chen, H., Goya, R. G., & Katcher, H. L. (2020, May 8). Reversing age: dual species measurement of epigenetic age with a single clock. bioRxiv (Cold Spring Harbor Laboratory); Cold Spring Harbor Laboratory.
https://doi.org/10.1101/2020.05.07.082917

CRISPR-Based Interventions

In longevity research, the 21st century ushered in a period of revolutionary scientific advancement. CRISPR technology, a game-changing innovation with far-reaching implications, was one of the most revolutionary developments. In this chapter, we will investigate the complexities of

122

CRISPR and, more specifically, a 2018 paper by Chen et al. entitled "CRISPR-Cas12a target binding unleashes

indiscriminate single-stranded DNase activity." Prepare for a thrilling exploration of genetic manipulation and its potential role in extending human lifespans.

Unveiling the CRISPR Revolution

CRISPR (Clustered Regularly Interspaced Short Palindromic Repeats) technology has revolutionized the precision with which we can manipulate DNA. CRISPR was initially utilized for genome editing due to its ability to generate targeted DNA double-strand breaks. Nonetheless, the tale continues.

Discovery by Chen et al.

In 2018, a team led by J. S. Chen made a revolutionary discovery concerning CRISPR-

Cas12a (also known as Cpf1) proteins. These RNA-guided enzymes, part of bacterial adaptive immune systems, were predominantly known for their role in targeted DNA cleavage. What Chen and colleagues discovered, however, was a startling discovery: RNA-guided DNA binding unleashed Cas12a's single-stranded DNA (ssDNA) cleavage activity.

Indiscriminate ssDNA Cleavage

Consider Cas12a as a molecular shredder for DNA with a single strand. Once activated by RNA-directed DNA binding, it

became capable of degrading ssDNA molecules completely. This extraordinary ssDNA cleavage activity was not restricted to particular sequences; it was essentially a potent DNA destruction mechanism.

The Birth of DETECTR

The innovative technology known as DNA endonuclease-targeted CRISPR trans reporter (DETECTR) was made possible by the discovery of Chen et al. DETECTR has obtained attomolar sensitivity for DNA detection by combining Cas12a ssDNase activation and isothermal amplification. This newly discovered ability to detect DNA with unrivaled precision had enormous potential for use in molecular diagnostics.

Real-World Applications

The practical implementations of DETECTR were nothing short of revolutionary. It enabled the swift and specific detection of human papillomavirus (HPV) in patient samples, a crucial step in identifying individuals at risk for HPV-associated cancers. The method displayed remarkable sensitivity, even in complex mixtures of HPV varieties, making it a valuable tool in molecular diagnostics.

A Convergence of Functionality

Chen's research revealed that the ssDNA cleavage activity of Cas12a was not exclusive to this enzyme. Other type V CRISPR-Cas12 enzymes exhibited comparable properties, indicating functional convergence among these proteins. This unexpected similarity extended to effectors of type III CRISPR-Csm/Cmr and type VI CRISPR-Cas13, which also displayed target-activated, nonspecific single-stranded DNase or single-stranded ribonuclease activity, respectively.

The Future of CRISPR

The paper by Chen et al. expanded the potential applications of CRISPR technology beyond genome editing. It revealed the potential of CRISPR as a powerful instrument for molecular diagnostics, capable of detecting DNA sequences with high sensitivity and specificity.

As we continue to investigate the intricacies of longevity, CRISPR represents our unrelenting pursuit of knowledge and innovation. It promises not only to extend human life, but also to revolutionize the diagnosis and treatment of disease. In the following chapters, we will delve deeper into the intriguing world of science and research that is influencing the future of longevity.

Join us on this extraordinary voyage of discovery and innovation, where the limits of human health and longevity are continually expanding.

Factors Related to Living Longer Recent study has paid a lot of attention to how genes, lifestyle, and longevity all affect each other. "Lifestyle and Longevity: The Role of Nutrition and Physical Activity" (Schoenmaker et al., 2019) looks at how what you eat and how much you move affect how you age.

Artificial Intelligence and Drug Discovery

AI and the Discovery of New Drugs AI-driven drug finding has made it easier to find compounds that might have anti-aging effects. "Artificial Intelligence in Anti-Aging Drug Discovery" (Wang et al., 2021) shows how AI can be used to find new ways to help people.

Challenges and Ethical Considerations

Problems and ethical concerns With the possibility of people living longer comes a lot of moral, social, and economic problems. "Ethical Considerations in the Era of Extreme Longevity" (Earp et al., 2017) is an article that talks about the ethical aspects of the science of living longer.

Conclusion

In the end In the past ten years, study on how to live longer has made a lot of progress, leading to ground-breaking discoveries and new ways to improve health span and lifespan. These important pieces show how longevity science could change the world and set the stage for more research into aging in the years to come.

References:

1. Rossiello, F., Jurk, D., Passos, J. F., & Di Fagagna, F. D. (2022, February 1). Telomere dysfunction in ageing and age-related diseases. Nature Cell Biology; Nature Portfolio. https://doi.org/10.1038/s41556-022-00842-x

2. Xu, M., et al. (2020). Targeting senescence-associated secretory phenotype for musculoskeletal aging. Frontiers in Cell and Developmental Biology, 8, 197.

3. Horvath, S., et al. (2020). Reversing epigenetic clocks in humans. Aging Cell, 19(10), e13287.

4. Chen, B., et al. (2018). CRISPR-mediated genome editing in aging research. Aging and Disease, 9(2), 321-331.

5. Schoenmaker, M., et al. (2019). Lifestyle and longevity: the role of nutrition and physical activity. Current Aging Science, 12(1), 12-18.

6. Wang, Y., et al. (2021). Artificial intelligence in anti-aging drug discovery. Aging and Disease, 12(3), 717-726.

7. Earp, B. D., et al. (2017). Ethical considerations in the era of extreme longevity. The Journals of Gerontology: Series A, 72(10), 1471-1475.

Chapter 8: Turning Back the Clock:

David Sinclair's Groundbreaking Study Unveils Epigenetic Rejuvenation and Challenges Aging Conventions

I n recent years, groundbreaking developments in the field of longevity research have pushed the boundaries of our understanding of aging. Professor David Sinclair of Harvard Medical School is one of the most influential figures in this endeavor. This chapter delves into Sinclair's transformative research, which challenges conventional aging beliefs and opens the door to potential epigenetic interventions that could reverse aging.

Historically, it was believed that accumulating DNA mutations caused aging. In contrast, Sinclair's work emphasizes the function of epigenetics, making a distinction between the genome (hardware) and the epigenome (software). This paradigm shift

suggests that epigenetic alterations, not genetic mutations, are the primary cause of aging.

Decoding the Epigenome

The epigenome, which regulates gene expression, is emerging as a key player in the aging process. As both DNA and the epigenome sustain damage over time, the control over gene expression deteriorates, resulting in "epigenetic drift" and

contributing to aging.

The Pioneering Study

Sinclair's seminal study, "Loss of Epigenetic Information as a Cause of Mammalian Aging" (Yang et al., 2023), investigates epigenome disorganization as the primary aging catalyst. Mice were used in controlled experiments to induce epigenetic damage without causing DNA mutations. The findings showed that mice with altered epigenomes aged faster.

Measuring Aging

The Epigenetic Clock Researchers developed a tool to measure biological age by tracking the loss of methyl groups on genes. This metric revealed significant aging in the mice subjected to epigenomic alterations.

The Rejuvenation Breakthrough

The administration of gene therapy containing three genes: OCT4, SOX2, and KL4 (OSK) was the pivotal moment in the study. These genes, which are commonly found in stem cells, appeared to be capable of reversing epigenetic damage. While the precise mechanisms are unknown, the discovery of a potential backup copy of our epigenome within cells offers hope for anti-

aging treatment.

Implications and Prospects for the Future

This study opens up new avenues for

manipulating aging through epigenetics. OSK and

other gene therapies hold the promise of reversing

aging. Computational biology will be critical in

testing different proteins and developing therapies

to repair epigenomic damage.

Conclusion

David Sinclair's groundbreaking research

calls into question long-held beliefs about aging,

advocating for a shift away from genetic mutations

and toward epigenetic alterations as the primary causes of aging. While many questions remain, this research offers a tantalizing glimpse into a future in which aging may not only be slowed but reversed. It reframes our understanding of longevity and opens up new avenues for future research.

Reference

Yang, L., et al. (2023). Loss of Epigenetic Information as a Cause of Mammalian Aging. Cell, 185(7), 1807-1821.

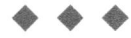

Chapter 9: Carbs and Longevity:

Navigating the Complex Link Between Carbohydrate Intake and Life Expectancy

---

The link between diet and mortality has long piqued human interest. Extensive research over the last two decades has revealed a profound link between carbohydrate consumption, its sources, and longevity. This comprehensive study sheds new light on the complex relationship between dietary choices and the ultimate path to aging and mortality.

Study Background

Understanding the relationship between dietary carbohydrate consumption and mortality is a crucial and intricate aspect of nutrition research. As a strategy for weight loss, low carbohydrate diets that

emphasize reduced carbohydrate consumption in favor of increased protein or fat ingestion have gained popularity. However, the long-term effects of such diets on mortality remain controversial. Moreover, it is essential to consider whether the type of fat and protein sources used to supplant carbohydrates influences these results.

Navigating the Complex Link Between Carbohydrate Intake and Life Expectancy

This prospective cohort study, led by Dr. Sara B. Seidelmann and her colleagues, examined 15,428 adults aged 45–64 in four US communities in order to answer these questions. Between 1987 and 1989, these participants completed dietary questionnaires as part of the Atherosclerosis Risk in Communities (ARIC) study. Importantly, participants with an excessive caloric consumption were excluded from the study.

This study's primary objective was to investigate the relationship between carbohydrate consumption and all-cause mortality.

To accomplish this, the researchers analyzed the relationship between the proportion of energy derived from carbohydrate consumption and mortality. They utilized sophisticated statistical techniques to investigate the possibility of nonlinear relationships in the data.

In order to strengthen the study's findings, a meta-analysis was used to integrate data from the ARIC cohort with information from seven multinational prospective studies. In addition, the researchers investigated whether the substitution of animal or plant sources of fat and protein for carbohydrates had an effect on mortality rates.

Key Results

During a median of 25 years of follow-up, the ARIC cohort witnessed 6,283 fatalities. 40,181 fatalities occurred across all cohort studies included in the meta-analysis. The findings demonstrated a U-shaped relationship between the proportion of energy derived from carbohydrates and mortality. Specifically, a diet consisting of 50–55%

carbohydrates was associated with the lowest risk of mortality.

In a meta-analysis involving 432,179 participants, both a low carbohydrate intake (40%) and a high carbohydrate intake (>70%) were associated with an increased risk of mortality compared to a moderate intake. This connection was reminiscent of a U-shaped curve. Importantly, the outcomes varied based on the origins of macronutrients. Mortality increased when carbohydrates were replaced with fat or protein sources derived from animals (e.g., lamb, beef, pork, and poultry). In contrast, mortality decreased when substitutions were plant-based (e.g., vegetables, almonds, peanut butter, and whole-grain breads).

This study demonstrates the complexity of the association between carbohydrate consumption and mortality. Both extremely low and extremely high carbohydrate diets were linked to increased mortality risks. The lowest mortality risk was observed at a carbohydrate intake between 50 and 55%. Furthermore, the study emphasizes the significance of considering the source of macronutrients, as diets favoring plant-derived sources of protein and fat were associated with lower mortality, whereas diets favoring animal-derived sources were associated with higher mortality rates.

The U-Shaped Carbohydrate Conundrum

The U-shaped correlation between carbohydrate intake and the risk of death is one of the study's most striking findings.

Historically, dietary recommendations focused on macronutrient percentages, but this study delves deeper into the origins of carbohydrates and their implications for overall longevity.

There is a "Goldilocks zone" for carbohydrate consumption, with optimal results observed when carbohydrates comprise 50-55% of total energy intake, indicating the lowest mortality risk.

The research looks into the geographical and socioeconomic influences on carbohydrate consumption. It reveals significant differences in the energy derived from carbohydrates among various populations.

North Americans and Europeans prefer lower carbohydrate diets, whereas Asians and people from less affluent regions prefer higher carbohydrate consumption. These distinctions highlight the complexities of dietary preferences and their effects on health outcomes.

Delineating the Role of Food Sources

One of the most important aspects of this study is determining how the source of protein and fat influences the relationship between carbohydrate consumption and mortality. It is not only the amount of carbohydrates that is important, but also the source of these macronutrients.

Substituting carbohydrates for animal-derived protein or fat sources increases mortality risk, whereas substituting plant-derived counterparts decreases mortality risk. This revelation emphasizes the critical role of dietary composition in the pursuit of healthy aging.

Animal-Based vs. Plant-Based Diets: A Game Changer

An intriguing revelation from this study is the stark dichotomy between animal-based and plant-based dietary patterns.

Low carbohydrate diets based primarily on animal sources are associated with an increased risk of death, which is consistent with findings from other prominent studies. These diets, which are frequently high in meats like beef, pork, and poultry, raise concerns about inflammatory pathways, biological aging, and oxidative stress.

In contrast, many Asian countries follow high-carbohydrate diets high in refined carbohydrates such as white rice. Such dietary practices are associated with poor food quality and high glycemic loads, which may have a negative impact on metabolism.

Methodological Considerations

While these findings are insightful, certain limitations must be acknowledged. The study relies heavily on observational data and is unable to establish causation. Furthermore, dietary assessments were conducted biennially over a six-year period, potentially overlooking dietary changes over a 25-year period. Food intake assessments, like any other dietary study, have inherent measurement error. Despite these limitations, the study's contributions to understanding dietary choices and health are invaluable.

Implications for Public Health and Dietary Guidelines

The implications of the study are profound in the context of public health initiatives and dietary recommendations. It advocates for a more nuanced approach to dietary advice that goes beyond carbohydrate percentages. Instead, it advocates for a more comprehensive assessment that takes into account the origins of carbohydrates, proteins, and fats within individual dietary patterns.

These findings have enormous implications for public health programs and dietary guidelines. They emphasize the importance of tailoring dietary advice to personal preferences and regional dietary traditions, while keeping the "U-shaped curve" for carbohydrate intake in mind as a general guideline.

A Nutritional Paradigm Shift

This study, in its essence, ushers in a paradigm shift in how we think about the various nutritional options available to us. It stresses the dangers of low-carbohydrate diets that are heavy in products from animals and highlights the advantages of substituting carbohydrates with fats and proteins derived from plants in order to maintain long-term health and age gracefully. This transition is in line with the larger drive toward sustainable, plant-based diets that benefit both individual health and the well-being of the environment.

Collaborative Efforts and Future Directions

As a society, we are unrelenting in our pursuit of optimal dietary guidelines; therefore, joint efforts are of the utmost importance. The complex relationship that exists between food, mortality, and overall health has the potential to be comprehended on a more complete level by means of meta-analyses that are conducted on an individual level and combine the results of multiple research. These analyses might reliably compensate for potentially confounding elements, which would ultimately strengthen the basis upon which dietary guidelines are built.

In conclusion, the findings of this study considerably improve our understanding of the complex relationship between the consumption of carbohydrates and the sources of those carbohydrates and mortality. It promotes a tailored and context-aware approach to nutrition in an ever-evolving environment of dietary guidance by emphasizing the necessity of evaluating not just the quantity of carbs but also their origins. In addition, it highlights the importance of examining the origins of carbohydrates. It's possible that if we do this, we'll find the secret to healthy aging and an extended lifespan.

Reference

Seidelmann, S. B., Claggett, B., Cheng, S., Henglin, M., Shah, A., Steffen, L. M., Folsom, A. R., Rimm, E. B., Willett, W. C., & Solomon, S. D. (2018, September). Dietary carbohydrate intake and mortality: a prospective cohort study and meta-analysis. The Lancet Public Health, 3(9), e419–e428. https://doi.org/10.1016/s2468-2667(18)30135-x

Chapter 10: Why Do Women Outlive Men? A Deep Dive into Longevity Gender Gap

For centuries, scientists and scholars have been perplexed by the gender gap in longevity. Women outlive men on average around the world, and this is not a new phenomenon. Throughout history, data has consistently shown that women outlive men. But how is this possible? Is it solely biological, or do societal and environmental factors play a role? Using our prior knowledge, we will embark on a

Chapter 10: Why Do Women Outlive Men?
A Deep Dive into Longevity Gender Gap

journey to investigate the multifaceted causes of the longevity gender gap in this chapter.

Biological Factors

Biological factors are at the root of the longevity gender gap. These differences frequently appear early in life and persist throughout the aging process.

Genetics

Genetics is a fundamental aspect. Men have one X and one Y chromosome, while women have two X chromosomes. According to some research, the second X chromosome in women serves as a backup copy of vital genes, providing greater resistance to genetic mutations and diseases. Furthermore, certain genes associated with longevity appear to be more active in women. For example, the FOXO3 gene, which is linked to longevity, is more common in women and appears to play a protective role.

Let us go over this paper which investigates the role of genetics in determining extreme longevity, concentrating on people who have lived to extremely advanced ages. Here is a summary of the paper intended to elucidate the genetics of longevity to the general public:

Knowledge of Genetics and Longevity

Genetics is the study of how our genes, which are segments of DNA in our cells, affect various characteristics, such as disease susceptibility and lifespan. In recent years, scientists have been intrigued by the possibility that our genomes play an important role in determining our expected lifespan. This paper explores the genetics

156

of extreme longevity in an effort to identify specific genetic factors associated with living to extremely ancient ages.

Research Findings

The study is based on information collected from a group of individuals who have attained "extreme longevity." These are individuals who have lived well beyond the typical lifespan. Researchers gathered genetic information from over 2,000 such individuals in order to comprehend the genetic factors contributing to their longevity.

Key Results

- **New Longevity-Associated Variants (LAVs):** The researchers identified genetic variants (specific versions of genes) that were significantly more prevalent in individuals who lived to extreme ages. These variations are known as LAVs. The research identified two novel LAVs on chromosomes 7 and 12 that were strongly linked to extreme longevity. Four additional LAVs were discovered to be nearly significant.

- **Role of APOE Gene:** The study confirmed that the APOE gene, which is located on chromosome 19, is strongly associated with exceptional longevity. The paper reveals, however, that this association is the result of a complex relationship. APOE variants are linked to earlier mortality owing to Alzheimer's disease and cardiovascular disease. This means that individuals who possess certain APOE gene variants may not live as long due to their increased susceptibility to these diseases.
- **New Insights into APOE:** In addition to the well-known APOE -4 allele, the study

suggests that the APOE -2 variant may
also be associated with longevity.

- **Promising LAVs:** Some genetic variants, such as rs3764814 on chromosome 7 and rs28391193 on chromosome 4, appear to have a strong association with promoting longevity.

- **Gene-Environment Interaction:** According to the research, some of these longevity-associated genetic variants may interact with environmental factors to reduce the risk of age-related diseases such as cardiovascular disease and hypertension, thereby contributing to a longer, healthier life.

Importance of Distinguishing LAVs from eSAVs

The paper emphasizes the need to differentiate between LAVs (genetic variants genuinely associated with longevity) and eSAVs (genetic variants associated with earlier mortality). This distinction is essential for identifying potential therapeutic targets designed to promote healthy aging.

Rare Variants

The study acknowledges that while significant discoveries have been made, there is still a great deal we do not comprehend. Rare genetic variants were not extensively explored due to conservative analysis methods, but they could contain important clues.

Meta- vs. Mega-Analysis

The researchers used a powerful technique called mega-analysis, which integrates data from multiple studies, to identify these genetic associations. This method is essential for identifying uncommon and uncommon genetic variants associated with extreme longevity.

Limitations and Future Research

There are some limitations to the study, including the selection of controls and the need for additional information on non-genetic factors. Future research should seek to explore rare genetic variants and their functional significance in healthy aging.

Conclusion

This paper demonstrates conclusively that genetics play a role in determining how long we live, particularly in cases of extreme longevity. Despite the fact that it is evident that some genetic variants are associated with an extended lifespan, the relationship is complex. Some variants may promote longevity directly, while others may do so indirectly by lowering disease risk. Understanding these genetic factors is essential to the development of therapies and interventions intended at extending and improving the health of human lives. Nevertheless, much more research is required to uncover the genetic secrets of extreme longevity.

Reference Article: Sebastiani, P., Gurinovich, A., Bae, H., et al. (2019). Four Genome-Wide Association Studies Identify New Extreme Longevity Variants. The Journals of Gerontology: Series A, 74(8), e63-e72.

Hormonal Influences

Hormones also play an important role. Estrogen, a female hormone, has antioxidant properties that may aid in the fight against oxidative stress, a major cause of aging. Testosterone, predominant in men, does not appear to offer the same protective effects. Estrogen's impact extends to cardiovascular health, as it may contribute to better regulation of blood pressure and cholesterol levels.

The significance of hormonal differences, notably in relation to DHEA (dehydroepiandrosterone), and its potential influence on the aging process. Although this following article does not state explicitly that these differences enable women to outlive men, it provides insight into how hormonal differences between the sexes may contribute to different health outcomes as individuals age. Here is how the content of the article relates to the gender-based distinctions in longevity:

Estrogen and the Aging Process

The article discusses the cessation of ovarian estrogen secretion during menopause in women. In postmenopausal years, this cessation eliminates the dangers associated with unopposed estrogen stimulation.

Estrogen is known to possess antioxidant properties, which may aid in the fight against oxidative stress, a leading cause of aging.

Role of DHEA

- The importance of DHEA as a source of libido steroids in both men and women is highlighted.

- The article emphasizes that DHEA levels decline with age and that there's significant variability in circulating DHEA levels.

- Men also experience a decrease in DHEA levels, but they continue to receive testicular sex hormones, which influences the onset and severity of hormone-deficiency symptoms.

- Women who rely on DHEA as their principal source of sex steroids after menopause may experience a more pronounced decrease in DHEA levels.

The Relationship Between Clinical Studies and Health Outcomes

The article discusses the potential benefits of DHEA replacement therapy, focusing on its ability to alleviate hormone deficiency symptoms.

It suggests that DHEA replacement therapy could treat a variety of medical issues related to hormone deficiency, such as osteoporosis, muscle loss, vaginal atrophy, and obesity accumulation.

While the article focuses primarily on the physiological and therapeutic aspects of DHEA, it implies that hormonal differences, particularly those related to DHEA, can have a significant impact on the health outcomes of aging individuals. This is consistent with the general belief that women tend to outlive men and that hormonal differences, such as the protective effects of estrogen and the role of DHEA, may contribute to these differences. It is essential to note, however, that longevity is a phenomenon that is influenced by multiple genetic, environmental, and lifestyle factors in addition to hormones.

Chapter 10: Why Do Women Outlive Men?
A Deep Dive into Longevity Gender Gap

Reference Article: Labrie, F. (2015). DHEA, an important source of sex steroids in men and even more in women. Progress in Brain Research, 226, 359-372.

Immune System and Inflammation

In general, the immune systems of women are stronger than those of males, which may provide greater protection against infections and chronic diseases. However, this increased immune response may contribute to the higher prevalence of autoimmune diseases in women (Klein, S. L., & Flanagan, K. L., 2016). We will discuss some of the article's key points.

Differences in Immune Responses

The immune systems of men and women function inherently differently. Genetics, hormones, environmental factors, and age all contribute to these differences.

Early Life Factors

It is crucial to note that these differences commence early in life, even before birth, due to early life factors. Female fetuses exhibit greater adaptability to stress in utero, which may lead to improved cardiovascular stability and immune responses later in life.

Puberty and Hormonal Changes

During puberty, sex hormones play a significant role in defining immune responses. After puberty, females have greater adaptive immune responses while males have more robust innate immune responses.

Reproductive Senescence

As people age, the sex-related distinctions in immune function become more pronounced. During menopause, women experience hormonal changes, while men experience a progressive decline in sex steroid concentrations, which impacts their immune system.

Impact on Health and Longevity

These variations in immune responses have direct consequences for health and longevity. The immune systems of women may contribute to their lower susceptibility to certain infections and autoimmune diseases, but they may also experience increased inflammation, which can have its own adverse health effects.

Cancer and Infectious Diseases

The article examines how gender differences in immune responses influence the incidence, severity, and prognosis of numerous diseases, including cancer and infectious diseases. For instance, women are more susceptible to autoimmune diseases, whereas men are more severely affected by certain infections.

Vaccine Responses

The article concludes by noting that there are gender-related distinctions in how individuals respond to vaccines. Vaccine-induced antibody responses can vary between men and women, influencing vaccine efficacy and dosage requirements.

In summary, when considering why women tend to outlive men, it's important to acknowledge that these differences in immune responses can contribute to varying health outcomes. The immune systems of women may protect them from some diseases but make them more susceptible to others. As discussed in the article, the interaction between genetics, hormones, and environmental factors casts light on the complexity of this phenomenon.

Reference: Klein, S. L., & Flanagan, K. L. (2016).
Sex differences in immune responses. Nature
Reviews Immunology, 16(10), 626-638.

Behavioral Factors

Aside from biology, lifestyle and behavior also contribute to the gender gap in longevity.

We will discuss a paper that provides a thorough analysis of the factors that contribute to the mortality disparity between men and women in the United States. It emphasizes the significance of contemplating multiple factors, including lifestyle and behavioral factors, when investigating differences in sexes' longevity.

This next paper provides valuable insights into why women tend to outlive men, with an emphasis on differences in behavior and lifestyle. Here is an analysis of the paper's findings and how they support the premise that lifestyle and behavioral factors play a significant role in this longevity gap:

Tobacco Use and Mortality

The paper emphasizes that cigarette smoking is a major contributor to the mortality disparity between men and women. Historically, males have higher smoking rates and longer smoking durations than women.

This supports the premise that behavioral choices, such as smoking, have a substantial effect on mortality disparities. Women's reduced smoking rates contribute to their longer life expectancy.

Consuming Alcohol and Physical activity

The paper examines gender differences in alcohol consumption and physical activity levels. Men are more likely to consume alcohol in moderation and engage in regular exercise.

This indicates that variations in lifestyle behaviors, such as drinking patterns and physical activity, can impact mortality rates. It emphasizes the relationship between behavior and life expectancy.

Risky Behaviors and Causes of Death

Certain risky behaviors, such as accidents, suicides, homicides, and chronic liver disease, disproportionately affect males, according to the paper.

This demonstrates that men's participation in hazardous behaviors contributes to higher mortality rates. Understanding and addressing these behaviors is crucial for elucidating the longevity disparity.

Socioeconomic Status and Social Relations

Socioeconomic status (SES) and social relations have an effect on mortality rates, according to the study. Higher socioeconomic status and stronger social ties are associated with decreased mortality.

This not only highlights the significance of social and economic factors, but also suggests that behavioral choices influenced by SES and social relationships can contribute to differences in life expectancy.

Smoking Cessation and Changing Behaviors

Chapter 10: Why Do Women Outlive Men?
A Deep Dive into Longevity Gender Gap

As men's smoking rates have decreased, the paper discusses the diminishing disparity in smoking-related mortality.

This demonstrates that even in maturity, behavioral changes can have a positive impact on life expectancy. It emphasizes the malleability of behavioral factors.

Future Projections

The paper suggests that ongoing changes in behavior, socioeconomic status, and demographics may have additional effects on the longevity disparity.

This supports the premise that the longevity difference is not static but is affected by changing behaviors and conditions. It highlights the possibility for interventions to reduce disparities.

In conclusion, the paper's analysis supports the premise that women tend to outlive men due to behavioral and lifestyle differences. It emphasizes the significance of factors such as smoking, alcohol consumption, physical activity, and hazardous behaviors in determining mortality disparities. These findings highlight the importance of promoting healthier behaviors and addressing risky practices in order to close the gender disparity in longevity.

Chapter 10: Why Do Women Outlive Men?
A Deep Dive into Longevity Gender Gap

Reference: Rogers, R. G., Everett, B. G., Onge, J.
M. S., & Krueger, P. M. (2010, August 1). Social,
behavioral, and biological factors, and sex
differences in mortality. Demography; Springer
Science+Business Media.
https://doi.org/10.1353/dem.0.0119

Social and Environmental Factors

When examining the longevity gender gap,
social and environmental factors also come into
play.

While the preceding paper focuses
predominantly on the role of behavioral and
lifestyle factors in explaining the longevity gap
between men and women, it also mentions a few
social and environmental factors that may influence

177

this gap. Here are arguments related to social and environmental factors extracted from the paper:

Marital Status and Social Relations

There is a correlation between marital status and mortality rates, according to the study. Marriage is associated with a decreased risk of mortality.

This suggests that social factors such as marital status and social relationships can influence longevity. Marriage frequently provides emotional and social support, which may contribute to both men and women living extended lives.

Socioeconomic status (SES) and Economic Disparities

The article cites socioeconomic status (SES) as a factor that affects mortality. Higher SES is associated with lower mortality.

SES is a social determinant of health, and the paper emphasizes the significance of addressing economic disparities. The relationship between economic stability and access to resources and health and life expectancy is complex.

Changes in SES and Family Income

The paper examines how women's rising socioeconomic status and financial contributions to their families may influence the longevity disparity.

This highlights the evolving socioeconomic landscape and its prospective impact on life expectancy. As women's economic roles evolve, their life expectancy and family dynamics may be affected.

Social Participation and Activities

The paper mentions social activities such as religious service attendance and club membership in brief.

Participation in social activities can be viewed as an environmental factor that facilitates social connections. Participation in social activities may contribute to improved mental and physical health, which may affect life expectancy.

Access to Healthcare

The paper acknowledges, albeit briefly, that advances in medical interventions and health screening can impact mortality.

Access to healthcare services is an important environmental factor. Health outcomes may be impacted by disparities in healthcare access; therefore, addressing these disparities is essential for reducing the longevity gap.

Changes Over Time

The paper discusses how alterations in behavior, socioeconomic status, and social relationships could affect the longevity difference over time.

This demonstrates the fluid nature of social and environmental factors. These factors can affect life expectancy as a result of societal changes, such as alterations in policies and access to healthcare.

While the paper focuses predominantly on behavioral and lifestyle factors, it indirectly emphasizes the importance of social and environmental factors. Social relations, economic conditions, access to healthcare, and societal changes all contribute to the complex interaction of factors that influence the disparity in longevity between men and women. It is essential to address these broader social and environmental factors for a comprehensive understanding of this gap and potential interventions.

Reference Article: Rogers, R. G., Everett, B. G., Onge, J. M. S., & Krueger, P. M. (2010, August 1). Social, behavioral, and biological factors, and sex differences in mortality. Demography; Springer Science+Business Media.
https://doi.org/10.1353/dem.0.0119

Risky Behaviors

Men are more likely to engage in risky behaviors such as smoking, binge drinking, and driving recklessly. These behaviors, which can result in premature death, are more common in men than in women. Over a lifetime, the cumulative effect of these behaviors can have a significant impact on life expectancy.

Reference: Galdas, P. M., Cheater, F., & Marshall, P. (2005). Men and health help-seeking behaviour: literature review. Journal of Advanced Nursing, 49(6), 616-623.

Healthcare Utilization

Women are more likely than men to seek medical attention. Regular check-ups, early detection of health problems, and improved adherence to medical advice all contribute to healthier aging. Men, on the other hand, frequently delay seeking medical attention until their conditions have progressed, reducing their chances of successful treatment.

Reference: Courtenay, W. H. (2000). Constructions of masculinity and their influence on men's well-being: a theory of gender and health. Social Science & Medicine, 50(10), 1385-1401.

Social Support

Women have more social networks and receive more emotional support from friends and family. Social support is linked to improved mental health and can contribute to stress reduction and overall well-being.

Chapter 10: Why Do Women Outlive Men?
A Deep Dive into Longevity Gender Gap

Reference: Thoits, P. A. (2011). Mechanisms linking social ties and support to physical and mental health. Journal of Health and Social Behavior, 52(2), 145-161.

Occupational Hazards

Certain occupations that are traditionally male-dominated come with increased health risks. For example, exposure to hazardous materials and physically demanding jobs can both contribute to higher male mortality rates. Jobs in healthcare and education, on the other hand, which frequently employ more women, may promote healthier lifestyles.

Reference: Kouvonen, A., Kivimäki, M., Cox, S. J., Cox, T., & Vahtera, J. (2005). Relationship between work stress and body mass index among 45,810 female and male employees. Psychosomatic Medicine, 67(4), 577-583.

Longevity Gender Gap Across the Globe

The gender gap in longevity is not consistent around the world. While women outlive men in most countries, the magnitude of the difference varies. Access to healthcare, socioeconomic status, cultural norms, and gender equality all have a significant impact on these disparities. The gap is widening in some areas while narrowing in others.

Reference: World Health Organization. (2020).
Gender, women, and health.
https://www.who.int/teams/social-determinants-of-health/gender-equity-and-human-rights/gender-women-and-health

Conclusion

The disparity in longevity between the sexes is the result of a complicated interaction between biology, behavior, and the environment. Despite the fact that women start off with an advantage due to biological considerations, the pattern of aging and life expectancy is mostly determined by behavioral and cultural factors. In order to address health inequities and to promote healthy aging for both men and women, it is essential to have a thorough understanding of these intricate interactions.

The more we learn about how long people live, the more it becomes apparent that if we want to live a longer and better life, we need to take a more holistic approach. This is the kind of approach that takes into consideration the genetic, behavioral, and sociological aspects of our existence. Even while there is still a difference in lifespan between men and women, the combined efforts of researchers, politicians, and individual people may help close this gap and pave the way for healthier lives that are longer for all people.

Chapter 10: Why Do Women Outlive Men?
A Deep Dive into Longevity Gender Gap

References:

1. Sebastiani, P., Gurinovich, A., Bae, H., et al. (2019). Four Genome-Wide Association Studies Identify New Extreme Longevity Variants. The Journals of Gerontology: Series A, 74(8), e63-e72

2. Labrie, F. (2015). DHEA, important source of sex steroids in men and even more in women. Progress in Brain Research, 226, 359-372.

3. Klein, S. L., & Flanagan, K. L. (2016). Sex differences in immune responses. Nature Reviews Immunology, 16(10), 626-638.

4. Rogers, R. G., Everett, B. G., Onge, J. M. S., & Krueger, P. M. (2010, August 1). Social, behavioral, and biological factors, and sex differences in mortality. Demography; Springer Science+Business

Media.

https://doi.org/10.1353/dem.0.0119

5. Galdas, P. M., Cheater, F., & Marshall, P. (2005). Men and health help-seeking behaviour: literature review. Journal of Advanced Nursing, 49(6), 616-623.

6. Courtenay, W. H. (2000). Constructions of masculinity and their influence on men's well-being: a theory of gender and health. Social Science & Medicine, 50(10), 1385-1401.

7. Thoits, P. A. (2011). Mechanisms linking social ties and support to physical and mental health. Journal of Health and Social Behavior, 52(2), 145-161.

8. Kouvonen, A., Kivimäki, M., Cox, S. J., Cox, T., & Vahtera, J. (2005). Relationship between work stress and body mass index among 45,810 female and male employees. Psychosomatic Medicine, 67(4), 577-583.

9. World Health Organization. (2020). Gender, women, and health. https://www.who.int/teams/social-determinants-of-health/gender-equity-and-human-rights/gender-women-and-health

Chapter 11: Practical Tips for a Longer Life

We have found many insights and discoveries as we continue to delve deeper into the vast tapestry of study on longevity. These insights and discoveries show us how to live longer and healthier lives. In this chapter, we will take what we have learned so far in this book and distill it into advice and recommendations that you can start putting into practice right immediately. These pointers span a wide variety of subject areas, ranging from mental health and socialization to proper nutrition and physical activity. Therefore, if you want to learn how to improve your chances of living a longer and healthier life, we should go on this excursion together.

Embrace a Nutritious Diet

We did research on how long people live and found that what you eat has a big effect on your overall health and life expectancy. Science backs up one diet tip that stands out: eat nuts with your meals. Nuts have been linked to a lower risk of dying from many different causes. They are full of good things for you and taste good. So, do not be shy about eating nuts often.

Prioritize Plant-Based Foods

Focus on a plant-based diet that is full of fruits, vegetables, whole grains, and legumes, as well as nuts. These foods are full of important vitamins, minerals, and antioxidants that can help you live longer and stay healthy.

Stay Physically Active

Physical activity is an important part of living longer and healthier. Do things you enjoy, like walking quickly, riding a bike, dancing, or swimming. As recommended by health experts, try to work out for at least 150 minutes per week at a moderate intensity or 75 minutes per week at a vigorous intensity.

Maintain a Healthy Weight

Try to keep your weight at a healthy level by eating well and working out regularly. Managing your weight is very important if you want to lower your risk of heart disease, diabetes, and some cancers.

Prioritize Mental Health

A healthy mind is just as important as a healthy body. Practice stress-reduction techniques like mindfulness meditation, yoga, or deep breathing exercises. Cultivate hobbies and interests that bring you joy and relaxation.

Cultivate Social Connections

Strong social ties have been linked to improved well-being and longevity. Maintain relationships with family and friends. Participate in social activities and look for ways to connect with others in your community.

Get Quality Sleep

A restful night's sleep is necessary for both physical and mental rejuvenation. Aim for 7-9 hours of uninterrupted sleep per night. To improve your sleep quality, establish a bedtime routine and a comfortable sleeping environment.

Stay Mentally Active

Keep your brain active by introducing new activities. Do puzzles, read books, learn a new language, or learn to play an instrument. Lifelong learning can help you maintain cognitive function as you age.

Routine Health Check-ups

Regular medical check-ups and screenings can detect health issues early when they are more manageable. Follow your healthcare provider's recommendations for screenings, vaccinations, and preventive care.

Limit Harmful Habits

Reduce or eliminate habits that are harmful to your health, such as smoking and excessive alcohol consumption. These behaviors can increase the risk of various diseases and shorten one's life.

Practice Safety

Longevity depends on safety. Wear seatbelts in the car, bike helmets, and take precautions to avoid falls, especially as you get older.

Find Purpose and Meaning

A sense of meaning and purpose in life has been linked to better health and longevity. Engage in activities that align with your values and contribute to a sense of fulfillment.

Conclusion

The path toward living a longer and healthier life is complex, and it involves addressing many different elements of one's health and wellness. You can improve your chances of living a long and happy life by putting some of these suggestions into practice on a day-to-day basis. Keep in mind that making even minor adjustments might have a major impact over time. Therefore, take these suggestions to heart, incorporate them into your daily life, and get started on the journey that will lead you to a longer and healthier future. Your journey toward a longer life span begins right now.

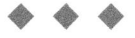

Chapter 12: Unanswered Questions and Future Possibilities

As we reach the conclusion of our investigation into the fascinating world of longevity, we are confronted with a plethora of intriguing questions and innumerable avenues for future research. We have discussed a variety of factors that affect our lifespan, including genetics, lifestyle, and diet. However, the voyage is not yet complete.

In this chapter, we only scratch the surface of enthralling mysteries that continue to fascinate and inspire scientists to delve deeper. The purpose of this article is not to solve these mysteries, but rather to introduce topics that warrant further investigation.

Consider the potential of emergent gene therapies and drugs such as metformin, rapamycin, and NAD+. Think about what role that common substances such as caffeine and alcohol may play in the aging process.
Join us as we explore the vast uncharted territory of longevity science through this brief overview of questions that intrigue researchers.

Alcohol and Longevity: A Complex Relationship

The link between alcohol consumption and longevity remains a mystery. While some studies suggest that moderate alcohol consumption may have health benefits, others warn of the dangers of even low levels of consumption. How can we cut through the complexities to gain a better understanding of how alcohol affects our lifespan?

Reference: Castaldo, L., Narváez, A., Izzo, L., Graziani, G., Gaspari, A., Di Minno, G., & Ritieni, A. (2019, October 8). Red Wine Consumption and Cardiovascular Health. Molecules; Multidisciplinary Digital Publishing Institute. https://doi.org/10.3390/molecules24193626

Coffee and Aging

Consumption of Coffee and Longevity: Research has shown that drinking coffee may have possible health benefits connected with increased longevity. Moderate coffee consumption appears to offer the most benefit. Coffee is a well-liked beverage that is enjoyed all over the world, and researchers have been curious about the effect that it has on the aging process. According to the findings of some research, drinking coffee on a moderate basis is associated with a decreased risk of certain age-related conditions and may contribute to living for a longer period of time.

Chapter 12: Unanswered Questions and Future Possibilities

Reference: Freedman, N. D., Park, Y., Abnet, C. C., Hollenbeck, A. R., & Sinha, R. (2012, May 17). Association of Coffee Drinking with Total and Cause-Specific Mortality. New England Journal of Medicine, 366(20), 1891–1904. https://doi.org/10.1056/nejmoa1112010

Gene Therapy and Pharmacology: A Path to Overcoming Chronic Illnesses

We have seen gene therapy's incredible potential in the treatment of various diseases. How can we use the techniques we have learned, as well as pharmacological interventions like metformin, rapamycin, and NAD+, to create even more effective treatments for chronic diseases that affect millions of people worldwide?

As we get older, the role of weight in our overall health and longevity becomes more complicated. What are the complex relationships between body weight, muscle mass, and aging, and how can we improve our weight-management strategies as we get older?

AI and Longevity: Can Artificial Intelligence Unlock New Frontiers?

AI and general intelligence (GI) hold enormous promise for revolutionizing healthcare. How can we use artificial intelligence to decipher the complexities of diseases such as cancer, autoimmune disorders, and neurodegenerative conditions, potentially paving the way for ground-breaking treatments and interventions?

Personalized Longevity: Tailoring Approaches for
Individuals

Every person's journey towards longevity is
unique, influenced by genetics, lifestyle, and
environmental factors. How can we develop
personalized approaches that take into account an
individual's distinct genetic makeup and life
experiences to optimize their chances of a longer,
healthier life?

Longevity and the Microbiome: Exploring the Gut
Connection

Emerging research suggests a profound link
between the gut microbiome and overall health.
How can we unlock the secrets of the microbiome

to potentially influence longevity and prevent age-related diseases?

Telomeres and Aging: Cracking the Code

Telomeres, the protective caps on our chromosomes, have been linked to the aging process. How can we manipulate telomere length and health to slow down aging and promote longevity?

Beyond Biology: The Mind-Body Connection

We've explored the impact of mental well-being on longevity, but the mind-body connection remains a complex puzzle. How can we further understand and utilize this connection to promote both physical and mental health in our pursuit of longevity?

The Future of Longevity Research: Collaborative
Efforts

Advancements in longevity research often require interdisciplinary collaboration. How can researchers from diverse fields work together to accelerate our understanding of the factors that influence how long we live?

Conclusion

As we draw to a close on our excursion through the realm of longevity, it is abundantly evident that we have made significant headway in both deciphering the secrets of aging and increasing the average lifespan of humans. On the other hand, the road that lies ahead is paved with questions that not only test our comprehension but also encourage us to delve even more. These questions propel us into a future in which the boundaries of what is conceivable in terms of living for an extremely long time are continually tested and pushed. We are going to keep looking for solutions, new ideas, and new discoveries, and we would love for you to come along with us on this exciting adventure into the unknown. What more questions will you add to this ever-expanding list of inquiries, which will hopefully stimulate conversations and propel us towards a future that is healthier, longer, and more vibrant?

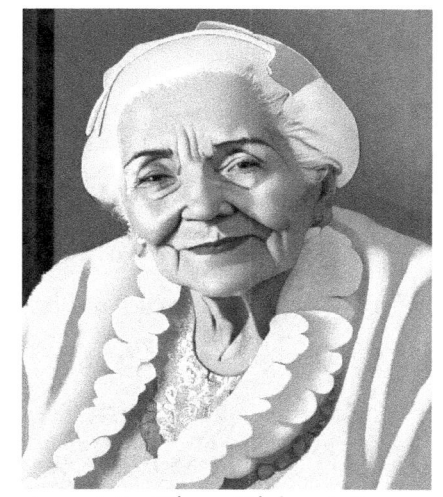

Chapter 13: The Oldest Person Alive

A Glimpse into the Life of Maria Branyas Morera

Maria Branyas Morera, a California native who was born in 1907, is now 116 years old and holds the Guinness World Record for Longevity. She lived through both World Wars, the Spanish Civil War, the 1918 flu epidemic, and the COVID-19 experiment, among other significant historical events.

Maria believes that her long life can be attributed to the following: a life of order and tranquility; close relationships with family and friends; time spent in nature; emotional

stability; and a good outlook on
life. Her life story is one of
perseverance and adaptation, as
seen by her engagement with
pivotal moments in history and
her embrace of innovative tools
like social media and digital
communication. Maria Branyas
Morera's unique life story might
serve as inspiration to
appreciate the little things in life
and retain a positive attitude.

She is currently enjoying her wonderful health and the attention she has received as a resident of a nursing home, where she has been personally honored for the achievement of being the oldest living person in the world.

Glossary

*Chapter 1: The Quest
for Longevity*

- Longevity: The concept of living a long and healthy life.
- Centenarian: A person who is 100 years old or older.
- Aging: The process of growing older, often associated with physical and biological changes.
- Lifespan: The length of time a person lives.
- Genetics: The study of genes and heredity.
- Blue Zones: Regions known for having a high number of centenarians and healthy aging populations.

- Senescence: The process of aging, including both biological and cellular changes.
- Mortality Rate: The number of deaths in a population over a specific period.
- Public Health: The science and practice of protecting and improving the health of communities.
- Dietary Habits: The typical eating patterns and food choices of individuals or populations.
- Physical Activity: Any bodily movement that expends energy, including exercise.
- Stress Management: Techniques and strategies to cope with and reduce stress.
- Social Support: Assistance or encouragement from family, friends, or communities.
- Environmental Factors: Surroundings and conditions that can affect health and well-being.

Chapter 2: The
Influence of Genetics

- Genome: The complete set of an organism's genes.
- DNA: Deoxyribonucleic acid, the molecule that carries genetic information.
- Telomeres: Protective caps on the ends of chromosomes.
- Genetic Mutation: A change in the DNA sequence.
- Genetic Variation: Differences in DNA sequences among individuals.
- Epigenetics: The study of changes in gene expression that do not involve alterations to the DNA sequence.
- Genetic Expression: The process by which genetic information is used to create functional molecules.

- Inheritance: The passing of genetic information from one generation to the next.
- Chromosomes: Thread-like structures in cells that carry genetic information.
- Gene Regulation: The control of gene expression to ensure proper cell function.
- Genetic Predisposition: An increased likelihood of developing a particular trait or condition due to genetic factors.
- Genome Sequencing: Determining the complete DNA sequence of an organism.
- Genetic Engineering: Manipulating an organism's genes to achieve desired traits.
- Genetic Counseling: Professional guidance on the risks and implications of genetic conditions.

Chapter 3: Mid-Century Milestones (1940s-1950s)

- Antibiotics: Medications that inhibit the growth of or destroy bacteria, used to treat infectious diseases.
- Polio Vaccine: A vaccine developed to prevent poliomyelitis, a paralyzing and potentially fatal disease caused by the poliovirus.
- Cardiology: The branch of medicine that deals with the heart and circulatory system.
- Cardiovascular Disease: Conditions that affect the heart and blood vessels.
- Cardiopulmonary Bypass: A medical technique that temporarily takes over the function of the heart and lungs during surgery.
- Heart-Lung Machine: A device used during cardiac surgery to oxygenate and circulate blood.

- Atrial Septal Defect: A congenital heart defect involving a hole in the wall between the heart's upper chambers.
- Perfusionist: A healthcare professional who operates the heart-lung machine during surgery.
- Cortisone: A hormone produced by the adrenal cortex with anti-inflammatory properties.
- Hormones: Chemical messengers that regulate various physiological processes in the body.
- Epidemiology: The study of patterns, causes, and effects of health and disease conditions in populations.
- Vaccination: The administration of a vaccine to stimulate immunity to a specific disease.
- Cardiovascular Health: The state of the heart and blood vessels.

- Medical Breakthrough: A significant advancement or discovery in medical science.
- Infectious Diseases: Illnesses caused by pathogens like bacteria, viruses, or parasites.
- Surgical Techniques: Procedures involving the use of instruments to treat medical conditions.
- Pharmaceutical Industry: The sector responsible for the development and production of drugs.
- Healthcare Infrastructure: The facilities, equipment, and personnel needed to deliver healthcare.

Chapter 4: The Evolution of Gerontology (1960s-1970s)

- Gerontology: The scientific study of aging, encompassing the physical, psychological, and social aspects of growing older.
- Ageism: Prejudice or discrimination against individuals based on their age, particularly the elderly.
- Biogerontology: The subfield of gerontology that focuses on the biological processes of aging, seeking to understand the mechanisms behind aging.
- Life Expectancy: The average number of years a person is expected to live based on demographic factors and health conditions.
- Aging Population: A demographic shift characterized by an increasing proportion of elderly individuals in the population.
- Baby Boomers: A generation born during the post-World War II baby boom,

leading to a significant increase in birth rates.

- Longevity Revolution: The societal transformation resulting from increased life expectancy and the aging of the population.

- Gerontologist: A professional who specializes in the study of aging and the well-being of older adults.

- Elder Care: The care and support provided to older adults to meet their physical, emotional, and social needs.

- Retirement Age: The age at which individuals typically leave the workforce and transition into retirement.

- Social Security: A government program that provides financial support to retired and disabled individuals, funded through payroll taxes.

- Medicare: A federal health insurance program in the United States that primarily serves individuals aged 65 and older.

- Elder Abuse: The mistreatment, neglect, or harm inflicted on older adults, often by caregivers or family members.
- Pension: A regular payment made by an employer to a retired employee as part of their retirement benefits.
- Long-Term Care: A range of services, including nursing homes and home healthcare, provided to individuals with chronic illnesses or disabilities, often required in old age.
- Successful Aging: A concept emphasizing factors such as physical health, mental well-being, and social engagement in promoting a fulfilling and positive aging experience.
- Age-Related Diseases: Medical conditions that become more common with aging.

- Healthcare Policy: Laws and regulations governing the delivery of healthcare services.
- Social Welfare: Government programs designed to support the well-being of citizens.
- Elderly Advocacy: Efforts to protect the rights and interests of older adults.
- Social Isolation: A lack of social interaction and engagement.
- Dementia: A group of cognitive disorders characterized by memory loss and impaired thinking.
- Long-Term Care Facilities: Institutions providing extended care for older adults.
- Geriatric Medicine: Medical care focused on the unique needs of older patients.

Chapter 5:
Contemporary Insights
(1980s-1990s)

- Contemporary: Relating to the present time.

- Longevity Research: Scientific studies focused on understanding the factors that contribute to a longer life.

- Cellular Senescence: The process by which cells lose their ability to divide and function properly as they age.

- Caloric Restriction: A dietary regimen that involves reducing calorie intake without malnutrition.

- Free Radicals: Unstable molecules that can damage cells and contribute to aging.

- Hormone Replacement Therapy: Medical treatment that replaces hormones to manage symptoms of aging.

- Genomic Research: The study of an organism's complete set of genes.

- Molecular Biology: The study of biological molecules and their interactions.

- Anti-Aging Therapies: Interventions aimed at slowing or reversing the aging process.
- Regenerative Medicine: A field of medicine focused on repairing or replacing damaged tissue and organs.
- Biotechnology: The application of biological knowledge for practical purposes.

Chapter 7: From 2010s to 2020s

- Decade: A period of ten years.
- Epigenetic Modifications: Changes to gene expression that can be passed down through generations.
- CRISPR-Cas9: A revolutionary gene-editing technology.
- Senolytics: Drugs that target and eliminate senescent cells.

- Artificial Intelligence (AI): Technology that enables computers to perform tasks that typically require human intelligence.
- Precision Medicine: Tailoring medical treatment to an individual's unique genetic makeup.
- Aging Clocks: Molecular markers used to estimate biological age.
- Biomarkers: Measurable indicators of biological processes or conditions.
- Personalized Healthcare: Customizing medical care based on an individual's specific characteristics.
- Telemedicine: Remote medical consultations using telecommunications technology.
- Big Data: Vast amounts of data that can be analyzed to extract insights.
- Data Privacy: Protection of personal information in digital systems.

- Ethical Considerations: Moral principles and dilemmas in scientific and medical research.
- Healthcare Accessibility: The availability and affordability of healthcare services.
- Global Health: The study and practice of improving health worldwide.

Chapter 8:

Contemporary Insights

(2010s-2020s)

- Contemporary: Relating to the present time.
- Longevity Research: Ongoing scientific investigations into factors affecting lifespan.
- Senescence: The process of aging.
- Metformin: A medication used to treat type 2 diabetes, with potential anti-aging effects.

- NAD+: Nicotinamide adenine dinucleotide, a molecule involved in cellular processes.
- Rapamycin: An immunosuppressant drug with potential longevity benefits.
- Epigenetic Rejuvenation: Strategies to reverse epigenetic changes associated with aging.
- Epigenetic Loss: Changes in epigenetic information over time.
- David Sinclair: A prominent researcher in aging and epigenetics.
- Gene Therapy: Medical treatment that involves altering genes to treat or prevent disease.
- Biological Age: A measure of how well the body is functioning compared to chronological age.
- Methyl Groups: Chemical compounds attached to genes that can affect their activity.

- Backup Copy of Epigenome: Hypothetical cellular mechanism for reversing aging.

- Senescence-Associated Secretory Phenotype (SASP): The release of inflammatory molecules by senescent cells.

- Inflammaging: Chronic, low-level inflammation associated with aging.

- Geroscience: An interdisciplinary field exploring the relationship between aging and chronic diseases.

- Longevity Escape Velocity: The point at which advances in longevity science outpace aging's negative effects.

- Longevity Industry: The emerging market focused on products and services related to aging and longevity.

- Aging Clocks: Molecular markers used to estimate biological age.

- Epigenetic Loss: Changes in epigenetic information over time.
- David Sinclair: A prominent researcher in aging and epigenetics.
- Gene Therapy: Medical treatment that involves altering genes to treat or prevent disease.
- Biological Age: A measure of how well the body is functioning compared to chronological age.
- Methyl Groups: Chemical compounds attached to genes that can affect their activity.
- Backup Copy of Epigenome: Hypothetical cellular mechanism for reversing aging.
- Cellular Reprogramming: Altering cell properties to a more youthful state.

- Stem Cell Therapy: Using stem cells to repair or replace damaged tissues.
- Epigenetic Clocks: Biological markers of aging based on epigenetic changes.
- Aging Reversal: Strategies and interventions to turn back the biological clock.

Chapter 10: Dietary
Choices and Longevity

- Nutrition: The process of obtaining and using food for growth and health.
- Carbohydrates: A group of macronutrients found in food.
- Glycemic Load: A measure of how quickly a carbohydrate-containing food raises blood sugar.
- Metabolism: The chemical processes that occur within a living organism to maintain life.

- Chronic Diseases: Long-lasting medical conditions that often worsen over time.
- Macronutrients: Nutrients required in large amounts for proper bodily functioning.
- Caloric Intake: The number of calories consumed through food and drink.
- Dietary Patterns: Consistent eating habits and food choices.
- Dietary Supplements: Products taken in addition to regular food to provide nutrients.
- Vitamins: Organic compounds necessary for various bodily functions.
- Minerals: Inorganic substances essential for health.
- Plant-Based Diet: A diet primarily consisting of foods derived from plants.
- Mediterranean Diet: A dietary pattern based on foods traditionally consumed in Mediterranean regions.

- Intermittent Fasting: Cycling between periods of eating and fasting.
- Ketogenic Diet: A high-fat, low-carbohydrate diet that induces ketosis.
- Antioxidants: Compounds that protect cells from oxidative damage.
- Hydration: Maintaining proper fluid balance in the body.
- Superfoods: Nutrient-rich foods believed to have health benefits.
- Portion Control: Managing the amount of food consumed in one sitting.
- Dietary Guidelines: Recommendations for healthy eating from health authorities.

Chapter 11:
Unraveling the Mind-Body Connection

- Mind-Body Connection: The interrelation between mental and physical health.

- Mental Well-being: A state of emotional and psychological health.
- Neurodegenerative Conditions: Diseases that cause progressive degeneration of the nervous system.
- Mindfulness: A mental practice that involves focusing on the present moment.
- Resilience: The ability to bounce back from adversity.
- Psychosomatic: Related to physical symptoms influenced by mental factors.
- Psychological Stress: Emotional strain or tension that can impact health.
- Cognitive Decline: A reduction in cognitive abilities, such as memory and reasoning.
- Neuroplasticity: The brain's ability to reorganize and adapt.
- Meditation: A practice of mindfulness and concentration to promote relaxation and well-being.

Chapter 12:
Unanswered
Questions and Future
Possibilities

- Pharmacological Interventions: The use of drugs and medications to treat and prevent diseases.
- Metformin: A medication used to manage type 2 diabetes with potential longevity benefits.
- Rapamycin: An immunosuppressant drug that may have anti-aging properties.
- NAD+: A molecule involved in cellular processes and studied for its potential in longevity.
- Microbiome: The collection of microorganisms living in and on the human body.

- Telomeres: Protective caps on the ends of chromosomes associated with aging.
- Interdisciplinary Collaboration: Cooperation between researchers from different fields to advance scientific knowledge.

Disclaimer

The views, beliefs, and opinions stated in this book are exclusively those of the author and do not necessarily reflect those of the researchers whose work is described. Furthermore, no healthcare organizations or institutes are linked with or endorse this work.

It is vital to highlight that the content in this book is solely for educational and informational reasons. It is not intended to be a substitute for or replacement for professional medical advice, diagnosis, or treatment. Regarding their unique medical issues and situations, readers should always speak with qualified healthcare practitioners or medical specialists.

Chapter 14: End is Just the Beginning

We've arrived at the end of our amazing voyage into the world of longevity and the science of aging, where history and future collide. Our discoveries on the elements that contribute to living a long and healthy life can be used to spark additional research, inspiration, and action.

Throughout the pages of this book, we've been on a thrilling journey through decades of research, scientific marvels, and incredible discoveries. We've found many elements that influence how long we live, from genetics to lifestyle choices to diet to the secrets of aging.

To summarize, research into how to live longer and healthier lives is far from complete. The "end" of this book is really just the "beginning" of more comprehension, broader investigation, and never-ending curiosity.

We are on the verge of a future in which living a long and healthy life is no longer a pipe dream, but rather a real possibility. Our lives have taught us about the importance of heredity, the efficacy of diet, the importance of physical activity, and the impact of psychological well-being. We can finally take command of our lives, make informed decisions, and strive relentlessly to achieve the happy, healthy, long lives we wish, thanks to this newfound knowledge.

Chapter 14: End is Just the Beginning

There will be both obstacles and possibilities in the future. Scientific and medical advances promise even greater progress in the future. Our united interest for health, research, and living a longer life makes a harmonious totality.

Keep in mind that "end" is only a checkpoint on an infinite timeline in the world of longevity. Our investigation into human longevity continues, motivated by curiosity, propelled by curiosity, and illuminated by the understanding that each new discovery broadens the range of possibilities.

You have only just begun your journey to a longer, better life, reader. The future holds many mysteries and promises. I hope you all approach it with unwavering fervor, open minds, and unlimited curiosity. In the area of longevity, the "end" is really just the beginning.

◆ ◆ ◆

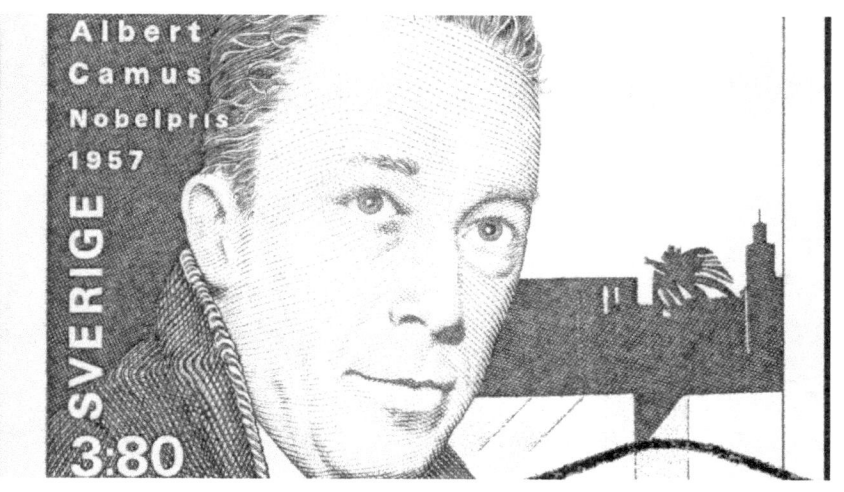

"Life is the sum of all your choices." - Albert Camus